# Practical
# Immunization

# PRACTICAL IMMUNIZATION

## George Dick

MD, DSc, MPH, FRCP, FRCPath, FIMLT

*Previously Assistant Director of the British Postgraduate
Medical Federation; Regional Postgraduate Dean to the
Southwest Thames Regional Health Authority, England;
Honorary Consultant at the Institute of Child Health, London;
Emeritus Professor of Pathology at London University.*

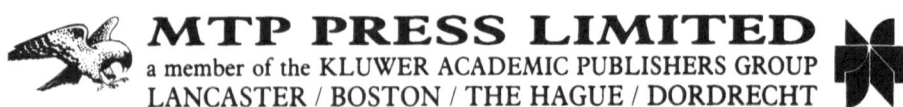

**MTP PRESS LIMITED**
a member of the KLUWER ACADEMIC PUBLISHERS GROUP
LANCASTER / BOSTON / THE HAGUE / DORDRECHT

Published in the UK and Europe by
MTP Press Limited
Falcon House
Lancaster, England

**British Library Cataloguing in Publication Data**

Dick, George
    Practical immunization.—[New ed.]
    1. Immunization
    I. Title
    614.4′7      RA638


Published in the USA by
MTP Press
A division of Kluwer Boston Inc
190 Old Derby Street
Hingham, MA 02043, USA

**Library of Congress Cataloging in Publication Data**

Dick, George.
    Practical immunization.
    Includes index.
    1. Immunization.   2. Communicable diseases—Preventive
inoculation.   3. Vaccines.   I. Title.   [DNLM: 1. Communicable Disease Control—methods.   2. Immunization.
3. Vaccines.   QW 800 D547p]
RA638.D52   1985      614.4′7      85–24058
ISBN-13: 978-94-010-8683-7      e-ISBN-13: 978-94-009-4926-3
DOI: 10.1007/978-94-009-4926-3

Typeset by Blackpool Typesetting Services Ltd., Blackpool, England

# Contents

# Preface

The development of immunization has been one of the most striking features in the control of infectious disease in the twentieth century. This book takes into account the need for a simple, concise account of immunization procedures not only in the UK and USA but also in other countries, and to this end a special chapter on immunization in developing countries has been included. Following two introductory chapters, there are nine chapters on various diseases and the vaccines that have been developed to combat them. In each of these chapters, a short discussion of the epidemiology of the disease and the history of immunization against it is followed by a description of the vaccine, its efficacy, contraindications to its use and future developments. These are followed by four general chapters on vaccines for travel, vaccines for selective use, passive immunization and immunization in tropical environments and the book concludes with a chapter on the smallpox vaccination and one on new vaccines.

The demand for this book follows the popularity of a series of articles on immunization which appeared in *Update*. These have been expanded and largely rewritten. I have drawn on many expert sources and have made an effort to provide a balanced and non-controversial opinion with a discussion of alternative procedures where indicated.

*Practical Immunization* is intended not only for the family practitioner but also for many specialists, particularly paediatricians, community physicians, and all those concerned with immigration procedures and with the spread of infectious diseases. Medical students, nurses and paramedical staff will also find much of value.

*George Dick*
*London*

# Acknowledgement

I wish to thank Dr Spence Galbraith and his colleagues at CDSC (PHLS) for providing some of the epidemiological data.

# 1
# Introduction

The prevention of infectious diseases depends on controlling or eliminating the source of infection, breaking the chain of transmission and on increasing the resistance of the individual to infection by general means or by immunization.

Many infectious diseases can be prevented without immunization, because once the natural history of the disease is understood, the source may be eliminated or transmission prevented. Thus, the prevention of rabies in the United Kingdom depends on controlling the importation of dogs and other animals from countries with endemic rabies (which now includes much of Europe). Similarly, psittacosis is prevented in man, not by routine immunization but by the control of imported parrots. When it was discovered in the 19th century that cholera and typhoid epidemics were regularly transmitted by faecal contamination of water, the provision of clean water supplies nearly eradicated these diseases from many countries without recourse to immunization. Again, yellow fever in urban areas was eliminated at the beginning of this century when it was discovered that it was transmitted by *Aedes aegypti*. All that was required was to stop the breeding of that particular mosquito.

## Socioeconomic conditions

The great reduction, and in some cases the virtual disappearance, of many diseases in some countries has been partly due to improved social conditions resulting in increased resistance to infection and reduction in transmission. Thus the mortality from measles in England at the beginning of this century was 30 per 100 000. In 1965, before the introduction of any vaccine, it had fallen to 0.1 per 100 000. Today the mortality of measles in many developing countries is of the same order as it was in Britain at the turn of the century.

In addition to the changes in incidence and mortality of some diseases which have apparently been brought about by changes in living conditions, there are other unknown factors which have affected the ecology of some diseases. Thus, scarlet fever was a mild disease when it was described by Sydenham in 1675, but in the middle of the 18th century it caused many deaths. It was again mild in the early part of the 19th century, became serious in the middle of that century but subsequently the death rate rapidly fell. Similar trends have been observed with other infectious diseases and there is no reason to assume that they are not still occurring. The vagaries in the mortality rates of infectious disease in the pre-immunization era should make one careful in attributing changes in the epidemiology of some disease to the result of specific treatment or immunization.

## Control of infectious disease

There is no doubt that the development of immunization has been one of the most striking features in control of infectious disease in recent years, but immunization is indicated only when the classic methods of control are impracticable or unsuccessful. For example, if cholera is introduced into the UK or the USA, there is no question of embarking on immunization, even if there were a highly effective vaccine, for cholera is unlikely to spread in these and other industrialized countries because of the high standard of public health practices.

There is no adequate way, other than by immunization, of controlling diseases which are transmitted by personal contact, such as the common respiratory or enterovirus infections. At the same time, just as surgeons must not forget the importance of asepsis in this antibiotic era, so physicians must not forget the importance of public health methods in the control of common infections. Thus isolation should not be written off as applying only to exotic diseases: contact between old people and children with respiratory diseases should be discouraged, small babies should be protected from being infected by siblings, and patients with influenza should be discouraged from battling to work until all their associates are infected. Good personal hygiene is still important in the prevention of disease. Whether we should use face masks during travel in crowded conditions to prevent the spread of influenza is difficult to decide. Masks have been used during influenza epidemics in the USSR and elsewhere, but there is no evidence of their value and indeed they might make spread of infection easier in some conditions by building up a high concentration of micro-organisms in the masks which would be readily transmitted during sneezing or coughing or when changing the masks.

## Immunization

Before considering immunization it must be shown that the disease in question is of sufficient severity, frequency or other importance to justify immunization against it. Nowadays no one would think of immunizing against plague or rabies in the UK for there is no risk of infection. There is little good reason for introducing mumps vaccine as a routine procedure, for the disease is usually mild, complications such as pancreatitis and orchitis are rare, and the prognosis of the common complications, namely meningitis and meningoencephalitis, is good. There may be a place for its use in certain circumstances (see page 129) but we must differentiate between selective and routine immunization. For example, while there is a good vaccine available against anthrax there is no question of making it routinely available; it should be used selectively for those at high risk.

If the infection is readily treatable there is seldom justification for immunization. I do not think that a very good case can be made for considering immunization against gonorrhoea, even if there were an effective vaccine. Is immunization the way to control that disease? Many would find it difficult to explain to 10-year-old children why they were being given a vaccine which implied acceptance, if not approval, of a certain social pathology. However, a gonorrhoea vaccine is something of the future. The natural disease does not produce immunity against reinfection and it will be difficult to improve on this. The control of gonorrhoea may depend on adequate treatment, education and better contact tracing, and on breaking the chain of infection rather than immunization.

In addition to having good epidemiological reasons for introducing a vaccine, there must be good evidence that the vaccine is effective and relatively safe. The risk of the disease in question must be greater than the risk of the immunization procedure. Serious reactions could be acceptable with a vaccine designed to prevent a disease with a high mortality and morbidity, but not with a disease with few serious complications.

It must always be remembered that there is nothing static about immunization procedures. They depend on the epidemiology of the disease at the time and place in question. What is right in Chicago may not apply to Ibadan.

There are two methods of achieving immunity: by active or by passive immunization.

## Active immunization

The best type of active immunization follows a clinical or subclinical natural infection. With many diseases this often gives lifelong protection at little or no cost to the individual or to the community.

Before measles vaccine was introduced, most children suffered a natural attack of the disease and measles was rare in adults because the body retains a 'memory' for many infectious agents which permits it to respond immediately if the agent is met again. The first contact with many infectious agents stimulates the production of antibodies which combine with and neutralize the agent or its toxins and/or sensitizes lymphocytes which are involved in cell-mediated immunity, but it also sets the stage for an immediate response when the infective agent is met again.

In the past, in countries without immunization programmes, and in many developing countries at present, most people have or had natural infections with all three types of poliomyelitis virus. This produced lifelong immunity but exacted a toll of about one paralytic case for every 1000 or so immunizing infections. With smallpox the cost in lives and disfigurements was so great that parents exposed their children to mild cases hoping that they would develop a modified infection and become immune for life. Before rubella vaccine was available this practice of actively exposing individuals to infection was in some places quite common and some parents held German measles 'tea parties' at which susceptible girls were exposed to infectious children in the hope of inducing an infection and lifelong immunity against rubella virus.

Whilst most people are naturally actively immunized for life against a host of infectious agents (many of which produce unrecognized infection), there are many infections which do not produce a durable immunity. The reason for this is that some infections are caused by multiple immunogenic types of the organism. Thus, while there is only one type of measles virus and of mumps virus, there are multiple types of influenza viruses which undergo antigenic changes every few years and thus make prevention exceedingly difficult. The short-lived immunity to some infections probably relates to the fact that they are very superficial and that there is thus little opportunity for the immune mechanisms to be stimulated.

## Artificial immunity

Artificial *active* immunization involves the administration of an antigen which stimulates immunity. These antigens may be in the form of live or inactivated micro-organisms or their products, e.g. toxins. Artificial *passive* immunization is achieved by injecting antibodies in the form of immunoglobulins.

## Live vaccines

Live vaccines consist of either an agent related to the causative micro-organism, as in the case of vaccinia, or of attenuated strains which are similar to the 'wild' strains in that they infect, replicate and immunize but differ in that they do not, or only rarely, cause illness.

Attenuation was first achieved by Pasteur with rabies vaccine, but really came into its own with the development of BCG (which is an attenuated bovine strain of *Mycobacterium tuberculosis*) and with the 17D strain of yellow fever virus (for use in areas where the insect vector could not be controlled) and then with poliomyelitis, measles, rubella and mumps virus vaccines. After a single dose of these live virus vaccines, immunity like that of a natural infection is produced. (The reason why three doses of oral poliovirus vaccine are given will be discussed later.)

The immunity produced by some vaccines is long lasting; with others, as with some natural infections, it may be short. Sufficient time has not yet elapsed to predict with certainty the durability of immunity with the live virus vaccines, which are now in common use, such as poliomyelitis, measles and rubella, but with most of them it appears that it will be long lasting. Live vaccines, as the name implies, consist of agents which are living. They infect and replicate and must be treated with respect. They are readily inactivated by light or when held for any length of time at room temperature and should therefore be stored in a refrigerator.

## Inactivated vaccines

Inactivated vaccines may consist of either suspensions of killed micro-organisms, e.g. whooping cough, typhoid, cholera and inactivated poliomyelitis vaccine, or of products or fractions of the micro-organisms such as the toxoids prepared from the toxins of *Coryne-bacterium diphtheriae* or *Clostridium tetani*, or of the diffusible fraction of *Bacillus anthracis* or fractions of viruses which contain a part of the micro-organism which is capable of inducing immunity as with one type of influenza vaccine or hepatitis B virus vaccine.

As with a natural infection, when a live vaccine is given, the replicating agent provides an antigenic stimulus over several days. The antibody response to inactivated vaccines is usually related to the quantity and potency of the antigen and so in order to produce an equivalent response to a dose of a live vaccine it would usually require a great weight of antigen which might produce severe reactions. Thus it has been found convenient to administer such antigens in divided doses. The first dose or doses 'prime' the immune response (primary immunization) and a population of memory cells are stimulated which provide a better and more rapid response (secondary response) when the antigen is met again. This secondary response occurs when further doses of the vaccine are given as well as when the natural infection is encountered.

While three properly spaced doses of inactivated vaccines are usually used to produce immunity, with some vaccines, e.g. inacti-vated poliovirus vaccine, this may be achieved with a single dose. If the individual has previously been exposed to natural infection with the micro-organism or to immunization, a single injection would usually be sufficient to recall or boost the immunity.

## Passive immunity

While active immunization lasts for a variable period and is often durable, passive immunity usually last for only weeks or months. It is achieved either naturally, by the passage of antibodies over the placenta and in colostrum which is the mechanism by which small babies are protected against many infectious diseases, or by the injection of immunoglobulins.

It will be recalled that in serum there are five classes of immunoglobulins, called IgG, IgM, IgA, IgD and IgE. IgG is the major one and accounts for about 80% of the total immunoglobulins. It is able to cross the placenta and diffuses readily into tissue spaces. It is responsible for neutralizing toxins (antitoxic antibody) and enhancing phagocytosis (opsonic activity). IgM is a macroglobulin and is the first immunoglobulin to appear in response to infections; it is particularly important in the agglutination and lysis of bacteria and in preventing bacteraemias and septicaemias. IgM does not cross the placenta or diffuse into tissue spaces. IgA appears selectively on mucous and epithelial surfaces and is obviously important in protecting the surfaces of the gastrointestinal and respiratory tracts from invasion by micro-organisms. IgE antibodies are involved in allergic conditions and the biological function of IgD is not yet fully established.

These immunoglobulins may be injected as (1) pooled human gammaglobulin which will contain antibodies to those diseases which are prevalent in the community; (2) specific gammaglobulin prepared (a) from individuals who are either recently convalescent from the disease in question, such as varicella/zoster, mumps etc or recently revaccinated or boosted, e.g. with hepatitis B vaccine or with tetanus toxoid or (b) now rarely, from animals, usually horses, immunized with, e.g. diphtheria toxin; (3) convalescent plasma which will contain IgM which is not normally present in the available immunoglobulins because of their method of preparation.

# 2
# Vaccines and Schedules

In this chapter, the types of vaccines which are generally available and suitable schedules for routine immunization will be outlined.

## Live virus vaccines (Table 1)

One of the main problems in the production of vaccines is to find a suitable substrate in which to grow the micro-organisms. While vaccinia virus for smallpox vaccine was grown on the skin of calves or sheep and the viruses for yellow fever and influenza in eggs, the virus vaccines which have been developed since the 1950s are grown in tissue cultures. These consist of layers of cells which have multiplied inside or on the walls of vessels which contain a nutrient medium. The tissue cultures are inoculated with virus which replicates in the cells and is released into the fluid phase of the culture and this fluid represents the vaccine.

**Table 1**  Live vaccines

| Vaccine | Sources of substrate for vaccine |
|---|---|
| Yellow fever | Chick embryo |
| Influenza | Chick embryo |
| Poliomyelitis | Monkey kidney or human diploid cells |
| Measles | Dog cells or chick embryo |
| Rubella | Duck, rabbit, dog or human diploid cells |
| Mumps | Chick embryo |
| BCG | Bacteriological media |

The tissues used for the vaccines must support viral replication to a reasonably high titre to make the production of the vaccine commercially acceptable and they must be free of any contaminating viruses or other agents. When monkey kidney tissue cultures were used to make vaccines, many people were inadvertently given a virus

(SV 40 – SV meaning 'simian virus') which was present in the monkey kidneys and as many as 60–80% of monkeys used were infected with one or other of these 'fellow traveller' viruses. Any tissue culture containing such contaminating viruses obviously had to be discarded. Some viruses, such as SV 40, are oncogenic in certain animals but there is so far no evidence that they have done any harm to individuals given vaccines which had been contaminated with them. The prevalence of these adventitious viruses in monkeys led to the use of tissue cultures from other mammals such as dogs and rabbits which could be more readily controlled, and to the further use of cultures from duck and chicken embryos. With the increased use of the latter, the number of adventitious viruses found in chickens continued to grow and methods had to be found for their elimination from flocks used for vaccine production. Until a few years ago, most batches of yellow fever virus vaccine contained a 'fellow traveller' chicken virus, but again there is no evidence of it having harmed those immunized with that vaccine.

The ubiquity of adventitious viruses in various mamalian tissues led manufacturers to use fully characterized standardized cells from animals or human fetal tissues which have been shown to be free from all detectable extraneous agents. Such cells are diploid and do not exhibit the properties of malignant cells. The early fears that such diploid cell lines might be carrying 'human cancer viruses' or cancer genes or the agents of slow virus infections have not been sustained.

The viruses selected for making live vaccines must be sufficiently attenuated so that they will not produce illness in vaccinated individuals, and yet must not be overattenuated or they may fail to multiply and immunize.

The method of attenuating viruses for vaccines is usually achieved by passage in non-human tissue cultures which tends to select mutants which grow better in the cells of a foreign host and become attenuated for man. The criteria of attenuation of strains suitable for vaccines were established for poliovirus vaccines and similar standards have been followed in the development of the newer vaccines. These strains must be genetically stable, and if they are excreted and transmitted to contacts they must remain attenuated. While tests of attenuation and safety are carried out in animals, the final evaluation of safety and effectiveness of all human vaccines must be in man.

9

The strain of the only live bacterial vaccine in common use, namely BCG, was attenuated by prolonged passage in suitable bacterial cultures.

## Inactivated virus vaccines

As far as inactivated virus vaccines are concerned, similar care has to be taken of the cultures used for growing the viruses, but the virus strains need not be attenuated because they will be inactivated by treating the culture fluids with formalin or other chemicals or by splitting the antigenic component from the virus particle. As a result of the inactivation processes, the chance of having a live extraneous agent in activated vaccines is obviously less than in live vaccines.

Inactivated bacterial vaccines are prepared by inactivating suspensions of the bacteria, by treating their toxins with formalin to form toxoids, or by preparing extracts of the bacteria.

Each vaccine, live or inactivated, has had its problems. These will be discussed under the individual vaccines, but in general, the problems encountered with live vaccines are mainly concerned with safety while those of inactivated vaccines relate mainly to efficacy. Both types of vaccines may sometimes present problems of untoward reactions.

**Table 2** Advantages and disadvantages of live and inactivated vaccines

| Advantages | Disadvantages |
| --- | --- |
| *Live vaccines:* | |
| Single dose given by natural route | Reversion to virulence dangerous if |
| Invokes full range of | there is natural spread to contacts |
| immunological responses, local | Viral interference may prevent |
| IgA as well as systemic antibody | infection by vaccine |
| production leading to possibility of | Inactivation in tropical climates |
| local eradication of wild viruses | |
| *Inactivated vaccines:* | |
| Potential of single dose vaccines | Given by injection |
| Adequate population coverage can | Multiple doses and boosters often |
| eliminate 'wild' viruses | needed |
| Stability | High concentration of antigens |
| | required |

The advantages and disadvantages of live and inactivated vaccines are shown in Table 2. There are qualifications which could be added, but the points form a useful basis for the subsequent discussions of individual vaccines.

## Schedules of routine immunization

Various schedules of immunization have been proposed, but only those recommended in the UK and in the USA will now be mentioned. Those suitable for developing countries will be discussed in Chapter 12. Schedules involving quadruple vaccine, as used in Canada, are outlined on page 59.

## United Kingdom

The schedule for routine immunization outlined in Table 3 is a general guide recommended by the Department of Health and Social Security in England. This schedule may not meet every case, but there are considerable advantages in having uniformity of procedure so that when children move from one place to another and change their doctors they will not be involved in a different course of immunization.

Since it is still necessary to immunize against diphtheria, whooping cough and poliomyelitis, it is desirable to provide the highest protection to the preschool child, in whom there is the highest risk of contracting or spreading these diseases. Although tetanus is rare in the UK, it is commonest in children, and it is convenient to include that vaccine with those of diphtheria and pertussis.

The starting time for the schedule outlined in Table 3 was previously more flexible but recently, in the hope of improving the efficacy of immunization against whooping cough, the majority of the Joint Committee on Vaccination and Immunisation of the DHSS have recommended that routine immunization with dip/tet/pert should commence at 3 months. Personally I think that there are good reasons for delaying immunization against diphtheria, tetanus, pertussis and poliomyelitis until the second half of the first year of life in children in industrialized countries. In the first place, with the exception of pertussis, infections with these diseases are rare in babies under 6 months of age in developed countries. Second, the presence of

Table 3   Recommended schedule for active routine immunization of normal individuals in the United Kingdom[1]

| Age | Vaccine | Interval | Notes |
| --- | --- | --- | --- |
| During the first year of life | Dip/tet/pert and oral poliovaccine (first dose) | | The basic course should start at about 3 months of age |
| | Dip/tet/pert and oral polio vaccine (second dose) | Preferably after an interval of about 6–8 weeks (at 4½–5 months of age) | |
| | Dip/tet/pert and oral polio vaccine (third dose) | Preferably after an interval of 4–6 months (at 8½–11 months of age) | |
| During the second year of life to puberty | Measles vaccine | After an interval of not less than 3 weeks | Ideally measles vaccination should be given in the second year of life: Any unvaccinated children should be vaccinated on entry to a playgroup, nursery school or school |
| At 5 years of age or school entry | Dip/tet and oral polio vaccine or dip/tet/polio vaccine | At least 3 years between last dose of basic course and boosting dose of dip/tet | |
| Between 10th and 14th birthdays | BCG vaccine | | Given to tuberculin negative children irrespective of whether or not a history of BCG at earlier age |
| All girls between 10th and 14th birthdays | Rubella vaccine | There should be an interval of not less than 3 weeks between BCG and rubella vaccination | All girls of this age should be offered rubella vaccine whether or not there is a past history of rubella |
| At 15–19 years of age or on leaving school | Polio vaccine (oral or inactivated) and tetanus toxoid | | |

[1] Data from Immunisation Against Infectious Diseases (1984). DHSS, London

maternally transmitted antibody (which the mother has acquired naturally or by immunization) masks the antigenic effect of certain vaccines given in the early months of life. It is sometimes possible to overcome this by giving larger doses of the vaccines, but this is unacceptable because of the reactions which might occur and their cost for routine use. Most maternal antibodies gradually disappear during the first 6 months of life: measles antibody can still have an inhibiting effect up to 12 months of age. Third, small babies are less immunologically mature than older ones. Although babies can respond to antigenic stimuli from a very early age, the immunity mechanism, particularly that of cell mediated immunity, is incompletely developed in the newborn. Finally, reactions to some vaccines may be more frequent in small babies than in older ones and are also less often recognized. Reactions to vaccines are unacceptable, not only because of the possible damage to the baby, but because the greater the number or severity of reactions, the larger will be the number of defaulters from completing the course of immunization.

Some say that if the start of immunization is delayed, the 'captive baby' will be lost. It is possible that some clinics are too rigidly organized, or have computer programmes which they do not care to change. With proper organization, I believe that immunization should, as far as possible, be the responsibility of the general practitioner who knows the baby and any contraindications to immunization which may exist in a particular child. With the present DHSS schedule using the triple antigen, the only good reason for starting immunization at 3 months and completing it as early as possible is the hope that this schedule will protect the *young* baby against pertussis of which, as yet, there is no evidence.

## *Spacing of doses*

The recommended interval between the first and second dose of dip/tet/pert and poliovirus vaccine is 6–8 weeks (Table 3). This is advantageous for oral polio vaccines (q.v.) as well as for dip/tet/pert and it is administratively convenient to give them at the same time. If the first and second doses of tetanus and diphtheria toxoids are closely spaced, then the second dose makes very little contribution to the ultimate antibody response. It appears that durable immunity will be obtained if the third dose is given at about 6 months after the second.

If the start of immunization is delayed till 6 months of age, an easy schedule for doctors and mothers to remember is – start at 6 months, second dose 6 weeks later, third dose 6 months later. Following this, no further immunization against diphtheria, tetanus, whooping cough or polio is required until school entry. At that time a booster of dip/tet and poliovirus vaccines, but not pertussis vaccine, should be given.

If immunization with dip/tet/pert is started before 3 months and if the intervals between the three injections are about 1 month, it may be necessary to give a booster of dip/tet/pert at 16–18 months. Those who support this latter programme usually fail to give the 16–18 months booster dose of vaccine. The 3-month starting date is also less satisfactory for immunization against poliomyelitis than commencing at about 6 months.

An interval of about 3 weeks should be allowed between giving two live vaccines (e.g. polio, measles, BCG and yellow fever). The reason for this is concerned with sorting out problems of reactions in some individuals rather than of any interference of the vaccine viruses.

## Interrupted programme

It must be appreciated that these proposed schedules are guidelines. It does not really matter if immunization is commenced a few days or weeks before the recommended age and it must be appreciated that a few weeks delay in the second or third doses is not vital. If one of the doses has been missed, then the subsequent doses should be given with the proposed intervals. Only if there are many months' interval between the first and second doses should consideration be given to restarting the basic course. If the immunization programme has been started at 6 months and the first two doses have been given, but the third dose has not been given at about 6 months later, then it is probable that if the third dose is given up to 12 months later, it will be effective in most cases. If only the first dose has been given at about 6 months, then two doses at about 6 months' interval should be adequate to complete the course.

Many children in the UK failed to receive pertussis vaccine in recent years and in order to ensure adequate coverage the schedule outlined in Table 4 is recommended.

**Table 4**  Schedule to complete immunizations where pertussis has been omitted

| Age | Vaccination status | Recommendation |
|---|---|---|
| Under 4 years | Dip/tet complete | 3 monthly doses of pert |
| 4–6 years | Dip/tet complete more than 3 years ago | Preschool booster of dip/tet/pert then 2 monthly doses of pert |
| Preschool (nursery school) | Dip/tet/pert incomplete | 1 dose dip/tet/pert. 2 monthly doses of pert |

## United States of America

The schedule which is recommended for healthy infants and children in the USA by the American Academy of Pediatrics is outlined in Table 5. Like the one recommended in the UK this is suggested as a guide which may require modification for certain individual or group requirements.

The Public Health Service Advisory Committee on Immunisation Practices (US Department of Health, Education and Welfare) recommends that immunization with dip/tet/pert should begin at 2 or 3 months of age or at the 6-week check-up, and that three doses should be given at 4–8-week intervals and a fourth dose approximately 1 year after the third. The primary course recommended for polio immunization is one of three doses, the first two doses preferably 8 weeks apart, and the third dose 8–12 months later. (The first dose is commonly given at the same time as the first dose of dip/tet/pert.) It will be noted that the age for beginning immunization is somewhat earlier than in the UK, but that a reinforcing dose of dip/tet/pert and oral polio vaccine is recommended at 1½ years of age.

## Hazards of immunization

Every vaccine carries certain hazards and can produce untoward reactions in some people. The importance of these reactions has to be weighed against the consequences of a natural infection. As noted, if the risk of being seriously incapacitated by a disease is high, severe reactions to the vaccine concerned are more acceptable than if the disease is mild and of little consequence. It is difficult to arrive at

**Table 5** Recommended schedule for active immunization of normal individuals in the USA[1]

| Age | Vaccine | Notes |
| --- | --- | --- |
| 2 months | Dip/tet/pert and oral polio vaccine | Suitable for breast fed as well as bottle fed babies |
| 4 months | Dip/tet/pert and oral polio vaccine | |
| 6 months | Dip/tet/pert and oral polio vaccine | |
| 1 year | Measles, rubella, mumps, tuberculin test | May be given at 1 year as combined measles – rubella or measles – mumps – rubella vaccines. Measles vaccine may be given at 6 months in places where measles frequent in first year of life. In such circumstances a repeat dose should be given at 1 year. Frequency of repeated tuberculin tests depends on risk of exposure and prevalence of tuberculosis. Initial test should be at time of, or preceding, measles immunization |
| 1½ years | Dip/tet/pert and oral polio vaccine | |
| 4-6 years | Dip/tet/pert and oral polio vaccine | |
| 14-16 years | Tet | And every 10 years thereafter |

[1] Data from *Report of the ·Committee on Infectious Diseases* (1974), 17th edition, American Academy of Pediatrics, Evanston, Illinois

precise estimates of the risks associated with some immunization procedures. Doctors are reluctant to consider an illness following immunization as being caused by something which they have recommended and have often persuaded the mother to accept for her baby. Local reactions will be obvious, but a complication of a severe nature occurring within 6-12 hours or 8-10 days after vaccination may not be considered as being possibly vaccine associated. It may well be an event which has occurred by chance following the immunization and is not in any way associated.

The known incidence of some of the reactions which follow immunizations may be of the order of 1:100 000, the physician may not have previously seen such a complication and may not associate it with immunization.

It is however important that practitioners should be aware of the known hazards which occur with the various vaccines. All serious reactions which follow the administration of any vaccine (whether considered to be caused by the vaccine or not) should be immediately reported. In the UK this notification should be made to the Committee on Safety of Medicines, DHSS, Elephant and Castle, London SE1 6BY, on the standard yellow card, and preferably also to the local district or community physician. In the USA reactions should be reported to the Center for Disease Control (CDC), US Public Health Service, Department of Health, Education and Welfare, Atlanta, Georgia 30333. Although CDC is principally a resource for local and State Departments it also offers direct and indirect services to practising physicians and hospitals in the USA.

## Contraindications

There are many myths and much confusion about the contraindications to immunization and conflicting opinions in comparing those listed in the product inserts of the vaccine producers, the ABPI, Data Sheet Compendium (Datapharm Publications Ltd, London), the British National Formulary and the DHSS (*Immunisation against Infectious Diseases*). These have recently been reviewed and assessed in a *Practical Guide to Immunisation* (Nottingham Child Health Unit).

The particular contraindications to individual vaccines will be discussed separately but the following apply to all vaccines.

Vaccines should not be given to children who are suffering from a febrile illness. The proposed schedules are sufficiently flexible to allow postponement of any of the doses and, as already noted, prolonging the interval between doses does not require starting the series again except if the interval between the first and second dose is more than 6 months. Minor infections such as colds and snuffles or a non-febrile rash should not be considered as contraindications and a reason for delaying immunization.

Allergy to eggs, unless extremely severe, is not a contraindication to immunization except with yellow fever vaccine. A history or family history of an allergic condition such as asthma or eczema is not a contraindication to any immunization: the only drug sensitivities which have to be considered are to neomycin and poliomixin in relation to measles vaccine. Live virus vaccines should not be given to individuals with immunological deficiencies or to those receiving immunosuppressive drugs, radiotherapy or parenteral steroids. Treatment with locally acting steroids, e.g. in inhalers for asthma, is not a contraindication. Live vaccines should not be given to those suffering from malignant conditions, e.g. lymphoma, leukaemia, Hodgkin's disease or other tumours of the reticuloendothelial system. Live virus vaccines should not be given routinely to pregnant women.

There is no contraindication to immunizing a baby who is being treated with an antibiotic.

## Reactions

Irritability, mild fever and malaise with some local swelling at the injection site for about 48 hours is quite frequent after the injection of vaccines. Parents should be warned that it is likely to occur. It is not a contraindication to further immunization.

Possible untoward events following individual vaccines are discussed separately but an anaphylactic reaction, although extremely rare, could occur after the injection of any vaccine. These reactions are manifest by wheezing, nausea and vomiting, and the more severe reactions which require immediate treatment with adrenaline consist of widespread oedema, particularly of the face, swelling of the tongue, severe bronchospasm, tachycardia, shock and collapse. Adrenaline (1:1000), syringes, needles and an airway should always be at hand at immunization sessions. The dose of adrenaline which must be given intramuscularly is 0.05 ml for under-1-year-old babies and 0.1 ml, 0.2 ml, 0.3 ml, 0.4 ml and 0.5 ml for children of 1, 2, 3–4, 5 and 6 years and over, respectively. The dose may be repeated if there is no improvement in 10 minutes.

If a child develops a severe reaction such as a convulsion, it must be considered as to whether the reaction is due to an intercurrent infection and has occurred by chance in relation to the immunization or is truly vaccine associated. The reaction should be reported and consultant advice obtained. Any really serious reaction is a contraindication to further immunization with the particular vaccine.

## Surveillance

We must be prepared to carry out continuous surveillance of immunization procedures. The usefulness of a vaccine may decrease with time, because of changes in the epidemiological pattern of the disease or in the formulation of the vaccine. The effectiveness of vaccine surveillance depends on the accuracy of reporting of the diseases and of vaccine complications and on serological surveys or other field trials of the vaccines in use.

# 3
# Diphtheria

Active immunization against diphtheria, which will be discussed in this chapter, is carried out with diphtheria toxoid. This consists of the toxin of *Corynebacterium diphtheriae*, which has been rendered non-toxigenic but has retained its antigenicity. This toxoid is usually given routinely as a triple vaccine which contains about 25 Lf* diphtheria toxoid, 5 Lf tetanus toxoid often absorbed onto a mineral carrier of insoluble aluminium salts and not more than $20 \times 20^9$ killed *Bordetella pertussis*. Passive immunization is considered in detail in Chapter 13.

## Diphtheria bacilli

There are three major types of *C. diphtheriae* – namely *gravis*, *intermedius* and *mitis*, so called because originally it was considered that *gravis* strains caused a more severe disease and higher mortality than *mitis* strains. This turned out to be incorrect. These strains may be toxic by virtue of a *phage* (the *tox + phage*) which they may carry. There are non-toxigenic *gravis*, *mitis* and *intermedius* strains of diphtheria bacilli which can cause a diphtheria-like disease and these and certain related species have been shown to be sensitive to toxigenic phages and then to produce toxin. In addition to these isolations of non-toxigenic strains from patients with a diphtheria-like disease, other species such as *C. ulcerans* and *C. haemolyticus* have recently been recovered from patients with membranous tonsillitis and an irritant rash but with no toxaemia.

---

* L means limit and f means flocculation: the Lf dose of toxin is determined by titration against the international antitoxin and the Lf unit is the amount of toxin which gives the most rapid flocculation with one unit of antitoxin.

# The disease

Diphtheria is characterized by fever and sore throat with a tonsillar and pharyngal or nasal exudate consisting of a tough fibrous membrane overlying a haemorrhagic and necrotic lesion. There is usually enlargement of lymph glands and the patient looks toxic. The diagnosis is confirmed by isolation of the bacilli from swabs rubbed vigorously over and under the membrane. Late in the illness motor paralysis and myocarditis may develop.

Diphtheria is essentially a carrier-borne disease and importations could occur silently and a focus of infection develop before the disease was recognized clinically. Many health workers will never have seen a case of diphtheria and if they do, it may well be atypical, for a *gravis* infection in an immunized person may look more like tonsillitis than diphtheria and non-toxigenic strains may produce a similar throat lesion but without toxicity. Outbreaks of group A β-haemolytic streptococcal pharyngitis must also be considered in the differential diagnosis and to a lesser extent other conditions giving a throat infection.

There is a wide range in the severity of diphtheria, and in the past the case fatality rate among children in developed countries has varied from 5% to 20%. Diphtheria infections with non-toxigenic strains are never fatal.

# History

In the 18th and 19th centuries deaths from scarlet fever were in excess of those from diphtheria, but by the late 1800s diphtheria was the most important cause of death in children (Figure 1). From 1870 to 1900 there was little change in the mortality, but since then there has been a continuous and unbroken decline. The reason for the drop in diphtheria mortality in the 1900s was presumably due to the introduction of antisera towards the end of the last century.

At the beginning of this century Behring and his colleagues in Germany showed that diphtheria was caused by a toxin formed by *C. diphtheriae*, rather than by invasion of the tissues, and that *C. diphtheriae* was capable of stimulating the production of a specific neutralizing antitoxin in the blood and tissue fluids on which immunity to the disease was largely dependent. Not only did these

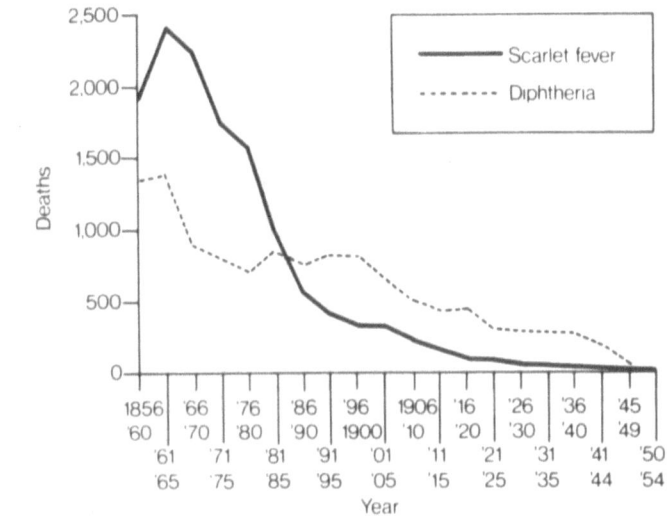

**Figure 1** Deaths from diphtheria and scarlet fever per million under 15 years of age, 1856-1954

observations lead to the development of antisera for treatment, which influenced the case fatality rate, but also to the development of toxoid for vaccines. The use of toxoid vaccines was pioneered by Park (1922) in the USA and by Glenny and Hopkins (1923) in England. In the USA they led to a drop from 100 000 cases with 15 000 deaths each year before 1925 to 307 notified cases with only five deaths in 1975.

It is surprising that the acceptance of this highly effective immunization procedure against diphtheria was so long delayed in Britain. The Ministry of Health had been advocating active immunization with toxoid since the early 1920s, but for the next 20 years the medical profession showed little enthusiasm for using the vaccine against a disease which in England and Wales was at that time killing 2000-3000 children annually. It can only be assumed that the failure of government propaganda to encourage immunization was due to a lack of confidence in the vaccine because there had been a few mishaps associated with its use in the USA and in some countries in Europe. Today it seems remarkable that the profession did not weigh these few mishaps against the thousands of deaths which were occurring every year (but cf. measles immunization, p. 88).

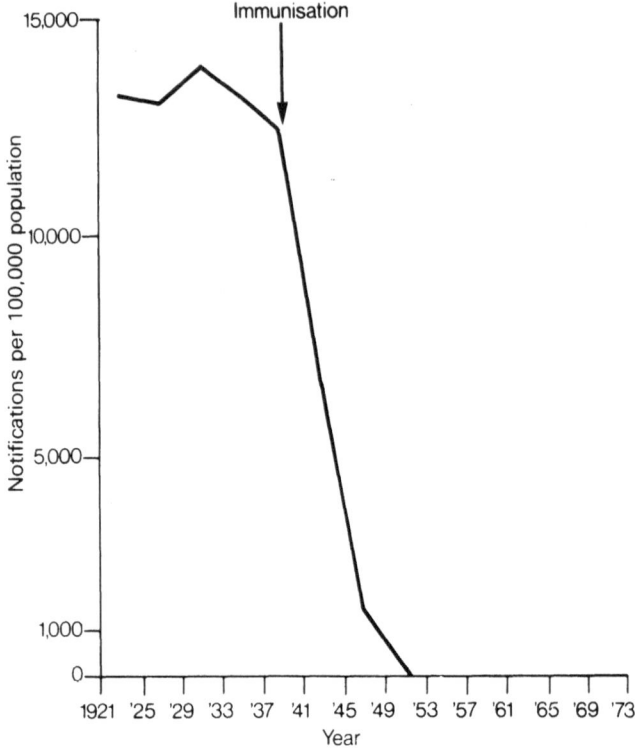

**Figure 2**   Notifications of diphtheria in England and Wales per 100 000 population

In 1941 extensive programmes of immunization were begun in the UK which were followed by a dramatic fall in the notifications and in the number of deaths from diphtheria (Figure 2). The disease has now virtually disappeared from the UK and from other countries with active immunization programmes.

In 1953 there were only 23 deaths from diphtheria in England and Wales (1 in 1 000 000 population) and Table 6 shows the number of deaths in recent years.

**Table 6**   Number of deaths from diphtheria – England and Wales

| 1954–58 | 1959–63 | 1964–68 | 1969–73 | 1974–78 | 1979–83 |
|---------|---------|---------|---------|---------|---------|
| 39 | 17 | 6 | 4 | 1 | 1 |

# Epidemiology

It was found in the early 1940s that diphtheria tended to disappear from communities in the UK where about 75% of the preschool and school children had been immunized. At the time, when these earlier immunization campaigns were under way, many adults were naturally immune as a result of childhood infections and it was calculated that the 'reproduction rate' of diphtheria was about four, i.e. each infected person could, in theory, give rise to an average of four cases. This rate depended on many factors but the disease must die out when the reproduction rate becomes less than one. This happened in the late 1940s in the UK when about 75% of the susceptible population were immunized. This 75% rate applies only to diphtheria in the epidemiological and social background of the 1940s. There is nothing magical in trying to achieve a 75% immunization rate in the prevention of other diseases. Poliomyelitis and measles have much higher reproduction rates and it is obvious that higher immunization rates (nearing 100%) will be required for their disappearance. On the other hand, smallpox disappeared from communities where only 50–60% of the population had been vaccinated.

The better implementation of immunization programmes has now eliminated the occasional outbreaks of diphtheria which centred around schools in the UK in the early 1960s. Now that there is little clinical diphtheria in the UK, diphtheria bacilli are rarely isolated and any which are recovered are usually non-toxigenic. Outbreaks which have occurred in the past 20 years or so have been located in hospitals for the mentally handicapped or have been introduced by immigrants.

In the USA from 1966 to 1970 there were 137 deaths from diphtheria, and only 43 between 1971 and 1975. The number of cases reported annually remains at between 150 and 800. All have occurred in localized outbreaks in different parts of the USA and many of these cases have been severe.

# Immunization

A history of having been immunized must not rule out a diagnosis of diphtheria.

Once diphtheria has ceased to be endemic in any country, it has been suggested that consideration should be given to abandoning routine immunization with toxoid. Although there are now high rates of immunization of children in the UK, the adult population is only about 20–50% immune as measured by the Schick test (see page 00). This could of course indicate a low sensitivity of the test, for although individuals are Schick negative when the blood contains less than 0.01 units of antitoxin per ml, those with lower levels may nevertheless be immune. There is some evidence to suggest that the immune rate in adults is falling, mainly because there are no pathogenic strains of *C. diphtheriae* circulating in the community which could boost the immunity. On the other hand, recent studies in Massachusetts have shown that titrations of 100 litre pools of adult plasma were found to contain 1 unit/ml of diphtheria antitoxin.

If there is a low rate of immunity in adults in the UK and there are no bacilli to boost artificial immunity, why does diphtheria not re-emerge when it is imported? Diphtheria may not have re-emerged in developed countries because the facility for spread of diphtheria among adults is much less than among children. Children are quantitatively better transmitters than adults both of bacteria and of viruses, and the method of spread of diphtheria may be less likely to occur among adults than children. If this is so, the reproduction rate in adults is presumably less than in children, perhaps only one or two. Therefore, nowadays quite a low rate of immunity in adults may be sufficient to prevent the spread of diphtheria if high rates of immunization are maintained in children. But there can be no reliance nowadays on carriers to maintain immunity and consideration may have to be given to periodic boosters to maintain protective levels of circulating antitoxins. There is at present no evidence that 'boosters' are required for adults in the UK, but there must be continuing surveillance.

Since diphtheria toxoid rarely causes any serious harm and since immunization can be carried out with little trouble with the combined vaccine, it would seem reasonable to continue routine immunization.

## Routine immunization

In addition to routine infant immunization with triple antigen, a reinforcing dose of dip/tet toxoid should be given at school entry (see Schedules, Chapter 2).

## High risk groups

Because of the efficacy of routine child immunization, those who are at high risk today in developed countries are not children but nursing staff and patients in homes for the mentally handicapped. Any patient admitted to such an institute and all nursing and other staff working in these homes should receive booster injections or a complete course of immunization if they have not previously received one. Reinforcing doses of toxoids are recommended for those working in countries where there is still a high incidence of the disease.

## Vaccines used

### Primary immunization of children under 10 years

Diphtheria toxoid by itself is rarely used for the routine immunization of children in the UK or the USA and in any event it is a poor antigen for primary immunization. It is usually combined in a dose of 25 Lf with tetanus toxoid (5 Lf) and both these components are often absorbed onto soluble aluminium salts along with *B. pertussis* vaccine which also acts as an adjuvant. In the UK the vaccine is usually given in three spaced doses in the first year of life (see Table 3) starting about 3 months of age, while in the USA the first dose is recommended at 6 weeks or older, followed by two further doses at 4–8 weeks' intervals and a fourth dose about 6 months after the third one (see Table 5). In the UK a booster of dip/tet is recommended at entry to primary school and, because of the risk of untoward reactions, the *B. pertussis* component is omitted from all combined vaccines for older children. A booster of dip/tet/pert at 4–6 years is recommended in the USA prior to entering kindergarten or primary school.

For reinforcement of immunity at school entry, either the absorbed or the fluid dip/tet vaccine may be used (the latter is not suitable for the primary course). A dip/tet vaccine is also available for the primary course. If there has been a reaction, other than a serious one, to the first dose of dip/tet/pert vaccine, then the adult vaccine described below may be given.

### Immunization of older children

In the past, in order to avoid allergic types of reactions which may be of every type, it was customary to carry out a Schick test on all

26

children over 10 years of age and on adults who required immunization. The reason for this was that the so-called purified toxoids not
only contain toxin–toxoid aggregates but also links of toxoid to other
diphtheria proteins and unrelated polypeptides that are present in the
culture fluids. In areas where diphtheria is endemic, many adolescents
and adults who have previously been infected clinically or subclinically with *C. diphtheriae* would develop hypersensitivity to the
products of *C. diphtheriae*, but this can also occur in infections with
non-toxigenic *C. diphtheriae* and other closely related corynebacteria
which are common commensals in the upper respiratory tract. It is
thus obvious that the frequency of hypersensitivity, particularly of the
delayed type, increases with age and is most frequent in countries
where the disease is endemic.

At the present time for the immunization of children over 10 years
and adults in developed countries (other than those likely to be
exposed to diphtheria in the course of their work), the Schick test is
omitted and the adult vaccine (containing only 1.5 Lf*) may be given
in a course of three doses at monthly intervals or as a single booster
dose. This adult diphtheria vaccine may also be combined with tetanus
toxoid (7.5 Lf) as a booster dose.

## Immunization of individuals likely to be exposed to diphtheria infection at work

The Schick test can not only identify susceptible individuals but also
those who are immune and might suffer severe reactions if given
toxoid in a 25 Lf dose. After injection of Schick test material, if no
circulating antitoxin is present (i.e. non-immunes) a red, slightly
haemorrhagic, reaction will appear within 48 hours at the inoculation
site and discoloration will persist for days. Immune individuals show
an immediate type of allergic reaction at the site of inoculation of
toxin and at the control site within minutes or a delayed tuberculin
response at both areas.

At the present time the classical Schick test has been generally
replaced in many areas by the direct measurement of serum antitoxin

* If the adult vaccine is not available the standard absorbed dip/toxoid vaccine may
be diluted, using all sterile precautions

levels. While in most cases adults who have had a primary course of immunization with diphtheria toxin can be boosted with the adult toxoid vaccine, those who consider that they have never been immunized should be Schick tested and appropriate action taken. A Schick titration may also be done in immunized health workers with a high risk of exposure to diphtheria to confirm their immunity. A level of 0.1 unit/ml is considered to be the level of antitoxin for adequate protection.

## Injections

The swabbing of a clean baby's arm before giving an injection is, I believe, purely ritualistic and if spirit is used it often causes stinging if not allowed to dry before the needle is inserted.

All vaccines should be administered from single dose ampoules by deep subcutaneous or intramuscular injection into the middle third of the deltoid or triceps muscle or into the vastus lateralis in the antero-lateral aspect of the thigh or the upper and outer quadrant of the buttock. It is of interest that there is some recent evidence which has shown that the response rate to at least one vaccine (HBV) is higher in hospitals using the arm rather than the buttock for the injections. It could be that vaccine deposited in the buttock is immobilized in fat.

## Adverse reactions

General reactions may consist of slight pyrexia, headache and malaise and a local reaction at the injection site representing hypersensitivity of the immediate, delayed or Arthus type (the latter associated with repeated boosters). All these hypersensitivity reactions seem to be more frequent in individuals who have a history or a family history of allergy. Very rarely there may be an anaphylactic reaction within minutes of the injection. Most health workers will never see such a reaction, but all those engaged in immunization should have adrenaline at hand (see page 18).

Neurological reactions following immunization with diphtheria toxoid are exceedingly rare: when they do occur following dip/tet/pert or dip/tet the component responsible is not usually identifiable. It must be remembered that reactions at first thought to be attributable to a vaccine may occur by chance.

With all absorbed vaccines, a hard module may persist at the site of inoculation for a week or two (the more obvious are usually associated with more superficial injections).

## Contraindications

Diphtheria vaccine should not be given to an individual who is suffering from an acute febrile illness. Considerations should be given to further immunization if there has been a *severe* reaction following the first dose. As already noted, the adult vaccine should be used in children over 10 years of age and in adults.

## Storage

The box of vaccine should be placed in a cool part of a refrigerator (2–10 °C) on receipt, and always stored there after use. Although some vaccines are supplied in rubber-capped bottles, individual ampoules are preferable for all immunizations.

## Community control

Community control of diphtheria depends on identifying and treating cases and immunizing both children and adults with two doses of dip/tet/pert, dip/tet or tet/dip not less than 4 weeks apart, and prophylactic treatment with penicillin or erythromycin if face to face contact occurred less than 7 days previously.

# 4
# Tetanus

Primary immunization against tetanus is carried out by routine immunization of babies with dip/tet/pert vaccine which contains 5 Lf of tetanus toxoid. This basic immunization can have no influence on the natural history of the disease, for *Clostridium tetani* is found in soil, house dust and in the faeces of animals and man throughout the world. The prevention of neonatal tetanus (tetanus neonatorum) is discussed in Chapter 12 and the prevention of tetanus following wounds with active and passive immunization in Chapter 13.

## *Clostridium tetani*

The prevalence of tetanus is dependent on the deposition of faecal material and can occur anywhere: the spores which are highly resistant can contaminate almost any substance including many items used in medicine. Like *C. diphtheriae*, *Cl. tetani* produces exotoxins one of which causes the disease.

When a wound is contaminated with the spores of *Cl. tetani*, they germinate in an anaerobic environment and the vegetative forms of the bacilli produce the toxin which reaches the nervous system by moving up the axons of nerves. The germination of the spores takes place most readily in devitalized necrotic tissue aided by calcium salts and pyogenic infections. *Cl. tetani* is not an invasive organism and the infection remains strictly localized. A natural attack of tetanus does not produce antitoxin in the blood and subsequent immunity, although it may prime the immune mechanism to respond to an injection of toxoid.

## The disease

The incubation period may range from 4–5 days to more than a month following infection through a wound which may be quite trivial, such as those caused by a thorn, nail or splinter. The toxin produces muscular spasm and contraction of voluntary muscles by inhibiting the release of inhibitory neurotransmitters from synaptic terminals in the c.n.s. Muscular spasms often first involve the area of injury and spasm of the masseter muscles (giving rise to 'lockjaw') and subsequently spasm of other muscles.

While classical tetanus is associated with dirty, lacerated or punctured wounds, 40–50% of cases of tetanus result from wounds which are so trivial that medical attention has not been sought. In as many as one third of the cases, there may be no detectable wound.

## History

The development of tetanus toxoid vaccine followed the pattern of that of diphtheria toxoid. Following the discovery, at the end of the last century, that serum of animals immunized with toxin was protective, numerous studies on its efficiency in man were made and its passive protective effect was established in studies of the wounded in World War I, but it was not till World War II that active immunization with toxoid was clearly established as being highly protective.

## Epidemiology

Tetanus is now relatively uncommon in industrialized countries because of basic immunization and the treatment of wounded persons. Those at high risk are manual labourers, road workers, mechanics, farm workers and gardeners and, as noted, the contaminated wound is often very trivial. Mortality from tetanus depends on the speed and efficacy of treatment, which should be carried out in special centres which have the necessary equipment and expertise. It is an important cause of death in rural tropical areas in South America, Africa and Asia.

In many developed countries deaths are reported from 'tetanus' or from 'injury complicated by tetanus'. Table 7 shows the reported number of deaths in England and Wales from 1955 to 1980. The actual figures may be higher because a death in which an injury has been complicated by tetanus may be notified as simply caused by an accident. With modern methods of treatment the case fatality rate today is probably about 20%, so that there may be about 100 cases of tetanus each year in England and Wales at present. Throughout the world, there are probably 100 000 deaths from tetanus each year; 30% of these are in the newborn which have resulted from contamination of the umbilical stump and these are preventable by immunizing mothers (see page 166).

**Table 7**  Reported deaths from tetanus – England and Wales – 1955–1980

| Deaths | 1955 | 1960 | 1965 | 1970 | 1975 | 1980 |
|---|---|---|---|---|---|---|
| Tetanus | 33 | 18 | 21 | 9 | 9 | 4 |
| Complicated by tetanus | 15 | 14 | 12 | 15 | 4 | 7 |
| Total | 48 | 32 | 33 | 24 | 13 | 11 |

Tetanus immunization was introduced in the UK in 1970 and its success has been reflected in the decline in deaths in the under-15-year age group (Table 8). The number of deaths in the 15–44-year-old (mostly due to sports injuries) has hardly changed over the years. In the 45-year-and-over age group, the increase in recent years, often following minor garden injuries, has been greater in females, presumably because many now-elderly males were immunized against tetanus during war service.

**Table 8**  Deaths associated with tetanus in England and Wales, 1969–1980 in various age groups

| Period | Age in years | | | | | | Total |
|---|---|---|---|---|---|---|---|
| | 0–14 | | 15–44 | | 45 and over | | |
| | No. | % | No. | % | No. | % | |
| 1969–74 | 22 | 18 | 38 | 31 | 61 | 50 | 121 |
| 1975–80 | 6 | 6 | 31 | 29 | 71 | 66 | 108 |

Although tetanus cannot be regarded as a major public health problem in developed countries, there should be even fewer cases with proper use of the preventive and prophylactic techniques available.

## Immunization

Routine infant immunization against tetanus is purely for the protection of the individual and has no community value because it cannot eliminate *Cl. tetani*.

Recent active immunization is effective in the prevention of the disease and if a person who has been actively immunized is exposed to the danger of tetanus, a reinforcing dose of toxoid at the time of injury will usually produce a rapid boost of circulating antitoxin which will afford protection. The objective of routine immunization in most developed countries is to provide a basic immunity in the entire population, which can be boosted at intervals throughout life and at the time of an injury suspected of being contaminated with *Cl. tetani*.

Individuals who have not been immunized as babies should be immunized as school leavers or as students or on entering employment. Those at high risk should be given a basic course of immunization and adequate boosters.

## Immunization of infants and young people

### Routine infant immunization

Tetanus toxoid is more effective when adsorbed on aluminium hydroxide. It may be given with diphtheria toxoid and *Bordetella pertussis* (the triple vaccine) or with diphtheria toxoid only (see p. 26). In general, the adsorbed toxoid produces a more durable immune response than simple fluid toxoid. The interval between doses for the basic course of immunization of infants has been discussed in Chapter 2.

Reactions to the tetanus component of the combined antigen are rare in infants and children and the reactions to dip/tet/pert are discussed in Chapters 3 and 5.

### Reinforcement of immunity

A reinforcing dose of dip/tet vaccine should be given at school entry and a dose of adsorbed tetanus toxoid vaccine is recommended on leaving school.

### Reactions

Reactions are rare but there may be some local swelling and pain at the site of inoculation. Children who have reacted to previous reinforcing doses may be given 0.1 ml of non-adsorbed simple toxoid intradermally which contains 4 Lf per 0.1 ml dose.

## Immunization of adults

For adults who have not been previously immunized, the adsorbed toxoid (10 Lf per 0.5 ml) is again preferred and three doses of vaccine should be given with an interval of not less than 6 weeks between the first and second dose and of about 6–12 months between the second and third. Persons who react to the first dose may be given a half dose of simple non-adsorbed fluid toxoid for the second and third doses. Alternatively, the course may be completed with simple fluid toxoid in 0.1 ml doses intradermally. The intradermal route seems to have about a three to five times adjuvant effect, so that a dose of 0.1 ml intradermally (i.d.) will have about the same antigenic effect as 0.5 ml given by the subcutaneous route. *The adsorbed vaccine must not be given i.d.*

While simple toxoid may be used for booster doses, all evidence suggests that the adsorbed toxoid produces a more durable immunity and should always be used for primary immunization. It is best to have only one preparation at hand for subcutaneous injection and the adsorbed toxoid is the one of choice. Three doses of fluid toxoid give a far less durable response than is obtained with two doses of the same toxoid adsorbed on aluminium phosphate.

## *Tetanus: duration of immunity and boosters*

The duration of immunity depends on the potency of the toxoid used and on the careful spacing of the primary and reinforcing doses. In the normal course of events, following the schedules described, boosters should not be required at intervals of less than 10 years and there is evidence which suggests that up to 30 years after primary immunization one dose of adsorbed tetanus toxoid is sufficient to stimulate the development of protective titres. Indeed, it may well be that an individual who has been immunized with potent vaccine as a baby and has had a reinforcing dose at school entry and school leaving will be immune for life, but this may not apply universally, e.g. in developing countries, perhaps as a result of malnutrition, babies may be less capable of responding to certain antigens and immunity may fall away faster in them than in babies and children in developed countries (see Chapter 12).

# Reactions

The incidence of reactions in adults is probably in the region of 1%. Reactions increase with age and with the frequency of reinforcing doses in those at high risk. There may be local swelling, pain and redness within a few hours of immunization which usually passes off in 3 or 4 days, but, sometimes what appears to be an Arthus type of reaction* develops about 10 days after inoculation, with considerable tenderness and malaise. Rarely there may be frank 'serum sickness' with onset about 10 days after inoculation. General reactions such as fever and malaise are uncommon, and the commonest type is urticaria with or without angioneurotic oedema.

Fluid toxoid is less reactogenic than adsorbed toxoid as well as being less antigenic. Individuals who develop reactions and require reinforcing doses should be given simple fluid toxoid intradermally. Any severe reactions should be reported in the UK to the Committee on Safety of Medicines, using the yellow card.

## Prophylaxis after injury

In conclusion, mention should be made of immunization in the prevention of tetanus following the receipt of a potentially contaminated wound. It is now generally accepted that the prophylaxis of tetanus following an injury primarily involves the use of tetanus toxoid. It seems clear that the recommended primary course of tetanus toxoid, with rare exceptions, supplies the necessary basic immunity so that boosters given at the time of injury will provide complete protection. (Because of medicolegal implications, antitetanus serum (ATS) continued to be used for many years after it was realized that it was harmful and indeed the number of deaths from ATS therapy in the UK exceeded those from tetanus.) Passive immunization with specific *human* tetanus immunoglobulin is required only for special cases.

---

* *Arthus-type rection*. When there is an excess of antigen, the complexes formed by antigen and antibody may be toxic to the tissues, for example, (1) in serum sickness where large amounts of foreign serum proteins (antigen) are circulating and antibody is beginning to be produced but is immediately combined with the antigen as it enters the circulation, or (2) when antibody is present in the blood and when high concentrations of antigen are injected into the tissue as in repeated injections of tetanus toxoids. The antigen–antibody complexes cause damage to the intima of small blood vessels

A simple guide to active and passive tetanus immunization at the time of wound cleansing and debridement, modified from that recommended by the Advisory Committee on Immunisation Practices of the US Public Health Service, is outlined in Table 9. This schedule presumes a reliable knowledge of the patient's immunization history.

**Table 9** Guide to tetanus prophylaxis in wound management*

| History of tetanus immunization | *Clean minor wounds* | | *All other wounds* | |
|---|---|---|---|---|
| | Toxoid | Immunoglobulin (human) | Toxoid | tet/ immunoglobulin (human) |
| *Dose* | | | | |
| Uncertain | Yes | No | Yes | Yes |
| 0-1 | Yes | No | Yes | Yes |
| 2 | Yes | No | Yes | No† |
| 3 or more | No‡ | No | No§ | No† |

\* Data from US Public Health Service Advisory Committee on Immunisation Practices (1977), MMWR, **26**, 29
† Unless wound more than 6 hours old
‡ Unless more than 10 years since last dose
§ Unless more than 5 years since last dose

It should be emphasized that all wounds are susceptible to tetanus and that they must be thoroughly cleansed of devitalized tissue and foreign material. For individuals who have had a complete course of immunization (four doses of toxoid), it is unnecessary to give booster injections more than once every 5 years (and probably 10) in wound management. If needed, 0.5 ml tetanus toxoid (adsorbed) should be given. If the wound is penetrating, extensive and very dirty and cannot be adequately cleansed or was sustained more than 6 hours previously, a dose of specific human antitetanus immunoglobulin should be given into the other arm. In wounds which cannot have complete debridement and where there are likely to be problems of healing, chemotherapy may also be used.

## Records

The most reliable and effective method of protecting the population against tetanus is to ensure that all are immunized. It would seem sensible that actively immunized adolescents and adults should carry a card recording their vaccination status.

## Contraindications

Booster doses of tetanus toxoid should not be given routinely at intervals of less than 10–15 years and at intervals of less than 5 years in wound prophylaxis. Repeated doses of toxoid may lead to hypersensitivity reactions which may be serious.

## Storage

The vaccine should be stored at 2–8 °C.

# 5
# Whooping Cough

Whooping cough or pertussis (*per* = very great: *tussis* = cough) is caused by *Bordetella pertussis* and is at present controlled by a vaccine of killed bacteria.

## *Bordetella pertussis*

In addition to *Bordetella pertussis*, called after Bordet, who with Gengou isolated this organism in 1906, there is another species of *Bordetella* called *B. parapertussis* which causes a mild pertussis-like disease. Whether *B. parapertussis* is truly a separate species or possibly a non-toxigenic strain of *B. pertussis* is not known. *B. pertussis* has several antigenic components, including a number of different agglutinogens (1, 2, 3, 4 etc) which vary in individual isolates, and some investigators consider that some of them must be included in a vaccine if it is going to be effective. The titres of the serum agglutinins which these agglutinogens stimulate are correlated with clinical protection from the disease. However, immunization with the vaccine, or infection with *B. pertussis*, does not always raise agglutinins and immunity may exist in the absence of demonstrable agglutinins. At the same time, infection does not take place in individuals who have serum agglutinins in high titre and the presence of agglutinins is indicative of the efficacy of a vaccine.

In addition to these agglutinins, there are several other antigens including the filamentous haemaglutinin (FHA) and the lymphocytosis-promoting factor (LPF) which seem to be important in stimulating protective antibodies and are important fractions of acellular vaccines at present under study.

## The disease

The onset of the disease usually presents as an afebrile cold which progresses with an increase in the number of coughing episodes, which become violent and paroxysmal. These are, to begin with, more common at night but later there is more coughing during the day with 20 or more episodes in 24 hours. The child makes an enormous effort to clear the respiratory passages of mucus, and when this is expelled there follows the whoop which is characteristic of the disease, and often vomiting. However, there may be no whoops and every child who whoops does not necessarily have whooping cough. Coughing may continue for months – the '100 days cough'. Complications may result from the violent coughing but bronchopneumonia and bronchiectasis complicating whooping cough appear to be things of the past in developed countries, presumably as a result of antibiotic therapy of bronchopneumonia associated with secondary invaders to which children with whooping cough are highly susceptible. Neurological complications such as seizures due to anoxia and encephalopathy may occur, but are rare. Severe infections and death are most frequent in the very young. But it is my impression that in many countries the clinical manifestations of whooping cough are much less severe now than they were in the pre-vaccine era, but parents in general are unaware of the nature of the disease.

## Diagnosis

No child should be labelled as having whooping cough unless the illness is bacteriologically proven or it has progressed for at least 3 weeks with severe paroxysms of coughing which often lead to vomiting. The diagnosis is usually based on the clinical picture (which is difficult in mild cases) and on the epidemiology of pertussis in the neighbourhood. The ability of laboratories to isolate *B. pertussis* from what appear to be typical cases varies enormously, but in any event by the time the clinical picture becomes suggestive the number of organisms in the respiratory secretions are decreased, making laboratory diagnosis difficult. Less than 50% of untreated cases will be positive after the third week. The best method for culture is from a Dacron swab of the nasopharynx. This is passed along the floor of one nostril. Rubbing of the swab on the nasopharynx may induce coughing which will enhance the chances of isolating *B. pertussis*. Alternatively a West's swab, which consists of a curved plastic tube housing a fibre tipped with Dacron, is introduced into the mouth and the curved end passed up behind the soft palate, and the swab is then pushed up into the nasopharynx and then withdrawn into the plastic tube. (I have never found this easy to manipulate in infants.) Higher recovery rates appear to be obtained using Augur suction to provide secretions. Some consider that the best method is to hold a bacteriological plate containing the special Bordet–Gengou medium in the front of the mouth of a coughing child. These 'cough plates' and other specimens must be taken to the laboratory immediately.

While failure to isolate *B. pertussis* may be a technical one, there are some viruses, e.g. adenoviruses, parainfluenza viruses and respiratory syncytial virus, which may give rise to an infection which is some respects may resemble that caused by *B. pertussis*. In some children other viruses may be present with *B. pertussis*, and it is possible that the severity of infection with *B. pertussis* may be potentiated by the secondary virus infection or vice versa. Some reappraisal of the aetiology of paroxysmal coughs in small children is required and physicians should make more use of the bacteriological and virological laboratory facilities available for confirmation of their diagnoses. They will thus become more skilled in the exact aetiological diagnosis of the conditions. It is always best to discuss the collection of specimens with the bacteriologist.

## Epidemiology

Whooping cough is spread by droplet infection and is maintained by person-to-person spread of *B. pertussis* from both clinical and sub-clinical cases. It may be transmitted by both children and adults.

In the UK and in the USA outbreaks of whooping cough have usually lasted for about 2 years and have occurred at intervals of roughly 3–4 years, but sporadic cases may occur at any time.

## Notification

Notification by general practitioners is, as a whole, erratic and inconsistent even for an individual doctor. However, it provides the most useful available index of the community effect of immunization (Figure 3).

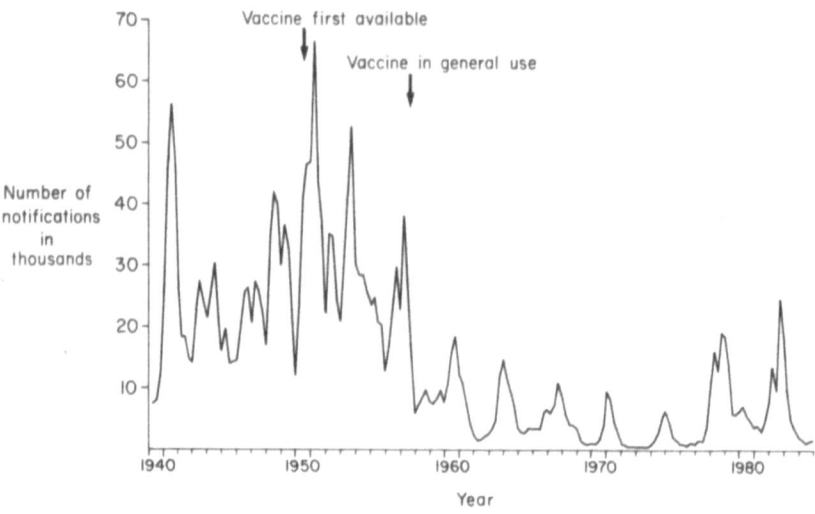

Source: Office of Population Censuses and Surveys

**Figure 3** Whooping cough notifications, England and Wales, 1940-85. (Prepared by CDSC)

While it is essentially a disease of infants and children, it may also infect adults in whom it may be a mild disease as a result of immunity following childhood infection or immunization but also because of a natural resistance of older people. While in the past it would appear that in developed countries the main source of infection of babies was from a sibling, nowadays much disease in infants and children may be of adult origin. While there is no evidence that pertussis is maintained as a 'carrier' disease, a continual source of infection may arise from subclinical, inapparent or mild infections.

## Mortality

For the past century there has been a steady decline in the recorded mortality from all infectious diseases in developed countries. In England and Wales until a few years ago (when measles vaccine became available), the decline in the mortality from whooping cough and that from measles had been very similar for 100 years (Figure 4).

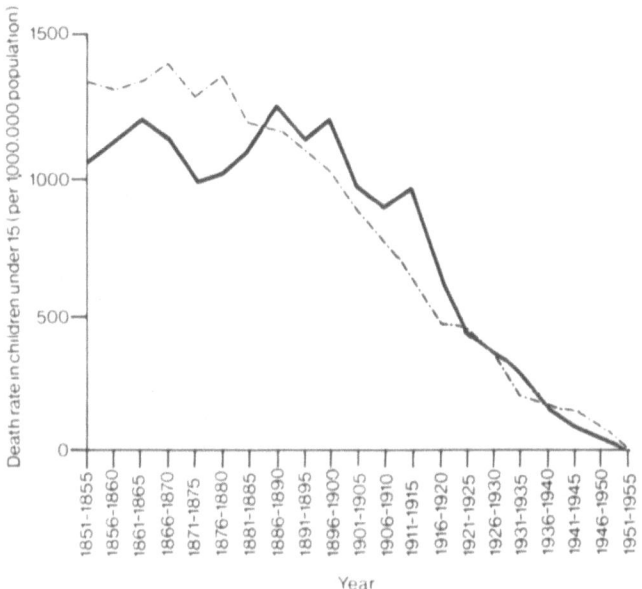

**Figure 4** Decline in deaths from whooping cough and measles (England and Wales). ————— = whooping cough; — · — · — = measles

The number of deaths began to fall long before there were vaccines or any effective drugs for the treatment of the diseases or their complications.

The mortality is much higher in the early months of life (Tables 10 and 11). It was suggested many years ago that as far as measles is concerned, anything which tends to postpone the age of attack will tend to make the disease less fatal. This also applies to whooping cough. It would seem that the reduction in family size, particularly in poor families, has been an important factor in the reduction of the mortality. In general, the mortality from whooping cough has been about 20 times higher in what was called social class V than in social class I. Infection is presumably brought to the family by the toddler/young schoolchild. Where there are large families with many small children and babies living in poor, crowded conditions, the disease causes more deaths than among small families living in better conditions.

When diphtheria vaccine was introduced the mortality from diphtheria showed an accelerated decline. On the other hand, when whooping cough vaccine was introduced no such dramatic drop in

**Table 10** Whooping cough deaths per 100 notifications (England and Wales)

| Year | Under 1 year | 1-4 years | 5-9 years |
|------|------|------|------|
| 1944–45 | 63.7 | 6.99 | 1.05 |
| 1946–49 | 42.6 | 4.07 | 0.40 |
| 1950–53 | 15.9 | 1.24 | 0.12 |
| 1954–57 | 8.8 | 0.55 | 0.09 |
| 1958–61 | 5.3 | 0.46 | 0.07 |
| 1962–65 | 9.2 | 0.60 | 0.04 |
| 1966–69 | 8.7 | 0.13 | — |
| 1970–73 | 8.2 | 0.24 | 0.14 |
| 1974–77 | 4.8 | 0.25 | — |
| 1078–81 | 2.7 | 0.09 | 0.03 |
| 1982–83 | 1.8 | 0.09 | — |

**Table 11** Whooping cough: deaths according to age in months, 1970–74, England and Wales

| Under 3 months | 3-5 months | 6-11 months | 12 months and over | All |
|------|------|------|------|------|
| 26 | 14 | 6 | 7 | 53 |

mortality was seen but the mortality continued its steady decline (see Figures 2 and 4). Vaccine does not appear to have had the influence which might have been expected on the decline of deaths. In previous chapters reference was made to the natural variations, over the years, of the severity of diphtheria and of scarlet fever. Could the fact that whooping cough has generally become a less fatal and a milder disease in recent years be related to a secular trend as well as to the use of vaccines?

## Vaccines

The routine whooping cough vaccines at present available consist of inactivated suspensions of *B. pertussis*. Like other vaccines prepared from whole bacterial cells (e.g. typhoid and cholera), whooping cough vaccines are not comparable in efficacy to the toxoid vaccines (such as those for diphtheria and tetanus) or to virus vaccines. However, although the presently-available vaccines may not always prevent pertussis, they do appear to reduce the severity of an attack and may modify infectivity within the family.

As already noted, the agglutinin response is not a direct measure of immunity and similarly the mouse potency test, which is the only available laboratory measure of potency, is not a direct or absolute measure of the efficacy of whole cell pertussis vaccines. At the same time it has been shown in clinical trials that the clinical efficacy of the vaccines correlated with the mouse potency test and the agglutinin response was related to protection from the disease.

Whooping cough vaccine is routinely given in combination with diphtheria and tetanus toxoids as a triple antigen or in quadruple vaccine.

## Age of immunization

The age of immunization against whooping cough varies from country to country (see Chapters 2 and 12). There is very little evidence that the vaccine is effective if given in the first few months of life (certainly very small babies are less efficient in their immune responses than older ones). Quite apart from the possible danger of more frequent reactions in smaller babies, mothers are nowadays loath to complete courses if their babies have been even mildly upset following an injection.

The schedules recommended in the USA and UK of starting immunization at from 2–3 months can give little direct protection to small babies. The main objective is the control of the disease in toddlers and preschool children (where there is the greatest morbidity) and thus reducing the chance of the infection being brought back into the family and spreading to small babies.

## History

Probably more research has been and is still being actively pursued towards the production of effective vaccines for whooping cough than for any other disease. As far as whole-cell pertussis vaccines are concerned field trials carried out in England in the 1940s by the Medical Research Council led to the manufacture of what appeared to be satisfactory vaccines. In ten trials where 4515 children were vaccinated and 4412 were controls, the average attack rate among their siblings with normal home exposure was 18% in the vaccinated and 87% in the unvaccinated group. With other less intimate exposure the attack rates were 8% and 38% respectively. One in five of the children in the vaccinated and unvaccinated groups were visited within 24–72 hours after each inoculation. In children immunized with vaccines which contained no alum, no severe local or general reactions were observed. Several developed a rise in temperature within 24 hours of inoculation and in some the inoculation site was red and swollen for 1 day to 2 days. However, in only a few were the reactions such that the mother objected to having the course of immunization completed.

Although there were variations in the potency of different batches of vaccines, even from the same source, the success of these trials set the stage for the introduction of immunization against whooping cough as a routine procedure in Britain in 1957. Following this, about 75% of children were immunized and there was a tenfold drop in notification (Figure 3).

Most countries which have introduced pertussis vaccine seem to have had little or no problem with their immunization programmes. In the USA cases and deaths from whooping cough declined dramatically following the introduction of vaccine in the late 1940s but in the UK the subsequent decline in morbidity was not what might have been expected with vaccines, some of which were claimed to give a protection rate of up to 90% in home exposures. Accordingly in the 1960s another field trial was carried out by the Public Health Laboratory Service, and it was discovered that as many as 56% of fully vaccinated children under 4 years of age developed whooping cough (confirmed bacteriologically), when exposed to pertussis in their homes. This was only a little less than the number of cases in an unvaccinated control group and it was concluded that some of the vaccine used before 1966 had less than the required potency of 4 iu* and this might account for the apparent vaccine failure. Alternatively, the serotypes of the prevalent strains of *B. pertussis* might have undergone changes and the new serotypes would not be represented in the vaccine. This explanation is not accepted by the majority of experts in Europe or the USA, who note that the decline in the incidence of

---

* iu = international unit(s)

whooping cough which many countries have experienced in the past few years has occurred in spite of using vaccines which did not contain serotypes of current strains.

In considering the epidemiology of whooping cough, one must consider the possibility of changes in the virulence of *B. pertussis*. When a considerable amount of the vaccine which was being used in the UK in the early and mid-1960s was relatively impotent why did the notifications not increase proportionally? (Figure 3). In Sweden the disease became very rare following the introduction of vaccine, but in 1970 following changes in the production methods, pertussis again became endemic; since 1974, however, it has become a mild disease.

While there is no evidence of changes in virulence of *B. pertussis*, although this is possible, it has been suggested that following the introduction of mass vaccination in Sweden in the 1950s, a large proportion of mothers were able to transfer immunity to their babies *in utero* or via colostrum. In the UK, although notifications of whooping cough fell dramatically after the introduction of vaccines, it appears that the lack of adequate control of vaccine potency led to continual sizeable outbreaks till the 1970s. Some vaccines which were issued in the mid-1960s contained a great excess of organisms $(29 \times 10^9)$ and only half the recommended number of antigenic units per dose. At the same time it was found that the reactions following the use of these vaccines was greater than was anticipated. The situation was remedied and vaccines were produced and standardized according to WHO requirements, but with the decline in the incidence of whooping cough there began to be some concern that the risk of reactions to the vaccine were too great and the public demanded that there should be some official investigation of serious vaccine complications, which led to the National Child Encephalopathy study.

## Immunization schedule

Whooping cough vaccine is routinely given as a component of the triple antigen dip/tet/pert and the schedules of immunization are discussed on page 11. It may also be given in a quadruple vaccine dip/tet/pert/polio. It has been suggested that if whooping cough is prevalent, three doses of triple vaccine may be given at monthly intervals, but such a course requires a booster dose of vaccine at 12–18 months of age.

Action to be taken if the basic course is interrupted is discussed on page 14. The presently available routine pertussis vaccine is not recommended for children over 6 years of age and reinforcing doses are not recommended after the basic course.

## Reactions

### Mild

The majority of infants and children develop some reaction following the administration of pertussis-containing vaccines. Local reactions consisting of swelling, redness and pain at the site of the injection are frequent, usually become apparent within a few hours after the inoculation and pass off within 12–24 hours. As noted, a small nodule may develop at the injection site but usually disappears within a week or two. At the same time the baby may be fretful, flushed, feverish and irritable or drowsy or may be off his feed for 24 hours. The local symptoms can be relieved with calamine or other cooling lotions and the general reactions with baby aspirin.

### Major

Reactions of persistent high-pitched screaming, collapse, convulsions and encephalopathy have been recorded. These reactions, although rare, were more frequent with the vaccines which were available in the 1960s and were more frequent in infants under 6 months of age. This is not surprising for, as noted, some of the vaccines in production at that time contained an excessive number of organisms, and increasing the number of organisms of a *B. pertussis* vaccine increases the frequency of reactions. One recent study in England did not confirm the observations of increased frequency of reactions in small babies, but this is not remarkable, for the vaccines were of different composition. Japanese experience suggests that the number and severity of adverse reactions associated with immunization may be reduced if vaccination is withheld till the child is older than 6 months (see page 11).

It was unfortunate that little official attention was paid to the observations which were made on certain vaccines which were in use in the early 1960s in N. Ireland.

## Neurological complications

It is not easy to establish an association between an immunization and a reaction unless it has a characteristic clinical picture and a definite time of onset following immunization, and preferably there should be a confirmatory laboratory test. There is no evidence that there is a specific clinical syndrome associated with present-day whooping cough vaccines.

*Convulsions and fits* which have been recorded following whooping cough vaccine are so frequent in small babies that they may occur by chance following an immunization and may not be causally associated. At the same time it has been shown that while there is no significant association between infantile spasms and pertussis immunization, the vaccine might trigger their onset. It has been suggested that convulsions associated with immunization are syncopal and extracerebral and that there is thus no evidence that they represent a transient encephalopathy, which in some children might not be transient but severe.

Public concern and lack of information prompted the setting up of a National Child Encephalopathy (NCES) study in the UK in 1976 which reported in 1981. In the NCES it was seen that children who were regarded as normal who developed neurological illnesses after immunization had a previous history of fits eight times more frequently than controls. It became clear from the NCES that there is a large background of potentially damaging neurological illness in infancy and early childhood of unknown aetiology which could occur by chance following immunization, but was not related to it. It was estimated that the risk of neurological illness following dip/tet/pert immunization from which most children made a complete recovery was of the order of more than one in 100 000 immunizations. The risk of encephalopathy was of the order of one in 310 000. While the study failed to establish a causal relationship of individual cases of neurological illness following dip/tet/pert or dip/tet immunization (which may be followed by similar neurological reactions), nevertheless it seems likely that a link may exist, but permanent damage of the c.n.s. following immunization with the presently available pertussis vaccines must be a very rare event.

If there were a 75% acceptance rate for pertussis vaccine a very approximate estimate of the number of children permanently damaged each year in the UK might be of the order of six to eight. The risk of a normal child developing a neurological illness after immunization with a pertussis-containing vaccine is about ten in 1 million and not all such reactions lead to *permanent* brain damage. The risk of immunization leading to permanent brain damage is about three in 1 million injections. It is well to compare this with some of the other risks to which our children are subjected, e.g. in 1979 one in 10 000 children of the 0–4 age group died from a road or home accident. More children died of whooping cough in 1977–9 than would have been severely damaged by immunization at that time.

In most other countries of the world the reactions following whooping cough vaccines seem to have been negligible. However, they have caused some concern in Sweden (where the use of pertussis vaccine was stopped in 1979) and in the Netherlands and in Denmark (where pertussis vaccine is no longer given combined with dip/tet toxoids but administered as a separate immunization).

Parents should be told that minor reactions are common but severe reactions are extremely rare.

In conclusion, it is clear that in the UK and in the USA the advantage of pertussis vaccine outweigh any risks associated with its use.

Any adverse reaction to the vaccine should be reported to the appropriate authority – in the UK to the Committee on Safety of Medicines, using the yellow card.

With all vaccines reactions can be greatly reduced by observing the contraindications.

## Contraindications

No child should be immunized in the acute phase of a febrile illness.

No child who had a *severe* local or general reaction to a preceding dose should be given a further dose of pertussis vaccine.

It is, at present, advised that a history of seizures, convulsions or cerebral irritation in the neonatal period or the presence of any neurological defects are contraindications but this advice may require reconsideration.

Children whose parents or siblings have a history of idiopathic epilepsy or of neurological defects require careful assessment as to the advisability of immunization.

There are no other contraindications; although allergy has been regarded as a contraindication to immunization, a considerable body of medical opinion no longer considers this to be so.

## Control of outbreaks

It might be possible to control an outbreak in some countries by a 'fire brigade action'. With an increased incidence of cases in any district, small babies might be immunized immediately an outbreak had started with a course of three injections of pertussis vaccine at 2–3-week intervals. The extent of such outbreak control programmes would depend on the local situation and it would have to be followed up later by routine immunization with the triple vaccine. In general, immunization of babies under 1 month is not recommended as a routine measure.

## Surveillance and acceptance

When routine whooping cough vaccine immunization was introduced in the UK there was no adequate surveillance system. If there had been, we would not have run into the problems which led to the setting up of the NCES.

In 1974 there began a sharp decline in the uptake of immunization against whooping cough because of some uncertainty about neurological reactions to the vaccine and this was followed by the largest outbreak of whooping cough since 1959 (Figure 3). The 1–4-year age group contained the children most affected by the decline in the vaccination acceptance rates which by 1978 had fallen from 75% to 30%. Because of this, about 1 200 000 children born between 1974 and 1976 were unvaccinated and the 1–4 age group showed a bigger increase in whooping cough than the 75% immunized in the 5–14 age group. Of interest was the large rise in the number of cases in the 25–34 age group, who were probably too old to be routinely immunized when young and were obviously at high risk if parents of unvaccinated young children. As might be expected, there was an interesting negative correlation between notification rates for Area Health Authorities in England and Wales and vaccine acceptance rates.

In general it has been pointed out that siblings tend to be immunized similarly and that if previous children in a family have fared well with the vaccine, the new child will do likewise; that 'the crucial decision is made about the first child'; and that 'efforts of those trying to increase the uptake ... are most profitably spent on the parents of the first born children'.

## The future

The whole-cell bacterial vaccine does not produce a durable immunity and this probably begins to drop away after about 2 years. This vaccine also has a degree of toxicity which has been discussed. In recent years, during inter-epidemic periods when the disease seemed to be less frequent in the community and in some areas mild, there has been a tendency to consider that the risks associated with the vaccine were greater than those of the disease, with a consequent decrease in acceptance and a subsequent increase in the incidence of pertussis. What is required is a vaccine producing a long-lasting immunity with no untoward reactions. Towards this end, efforts have been made to develop acellular vaccines.

Experimental acellular vaccines containing the FHA and LPF protective antigens (page 38) have been studied, and methods could be developed to standardize them accurately.

There is now some evidence which indicates that colostrum from naturally infected mothers contains protective antibodies and the immunization of mothers with potent non-reactogenic acellular vaccines might be a method of protecting babies at the most critical period in the first few months of life. At the same time the presence of such antibody in babies born of naturally immune or immunized mothers may inhibit their response to their immunization under 6 months of age, which is similar to the inhibitory effect of passive antibody to diphtheria. There are many laboratory and epidemiological problems to consider before pertussis is adequately controlled and a vaccine is available for all people which is both safe and effective in preventing both infection and disease.

# 6
# Poliomyelitis

Poliomyelitis is caused by a virus of the enterovirus group and is controlled by live oral poliovirus vaccine or by inactivated poliovirus vaccine.

## Polioviruses

Poliovirus belongs to the enterovirus group of picornaviruses (pico = small, RNA = ribonucleic acid). There are a large number of enteroviruses which are transient inhabitants of the human alimentary tract. They grow in tissue cultures and may be isolated from faeces, throat secretions and blood. There are three types of poliovirus - 1, 2 and 3. Poliovirus particles are 28 nm in diameter. They have a very limited host range but most strains will infect man, monkeys and chimpanzees. The three types show a certain amount of immunological cross-reaction. Two type specific antigens can be identified in poliovirus preparations - the N (native form) or D antigen and the H (heated) one. The N form represents full virus particles containing RNA and the H form empty particles.

## The disease

The disease is now very uncommon in developed countries because of the widespread use of vaccines. At the onset, there is mild fever and headache which may improve in a few days and there may be no further signs and symptoms (the minor illness), but it may progress to an illness with fever, muscle pains, headache and neck stiffness (aseptic meningitis) and to paralysis (paralytic poliomyelitis). The paralysis is typically flaccid, asymmetrical and of abrupt onset, usually involving the leg(s) and/or arm(s). There are rarely any sensory defects and no progression of symptoms after 3 days. (Other enteroviruses such as ECHO and Coxsackie viruses can cause illness simulating paralytic poliomyelitis.)

# History

Although poliomyelitis had been endemic for centuries it was not till about 80 years ago that it became an epidemic disease, first in Scandinavia and later in the USA where regular epidemics occurred from the early 1900s until the mid-1950s when immunization was introduced.

In the UK, about the beginning of this century, as in the earlier outbreaks in the USA, poliomyelitis was essentially 'infantile paralysis' and in one of these epidemics, for example, in Bristol in 1909, 80% of the 37 paralytic cases occurred in children under 3 years

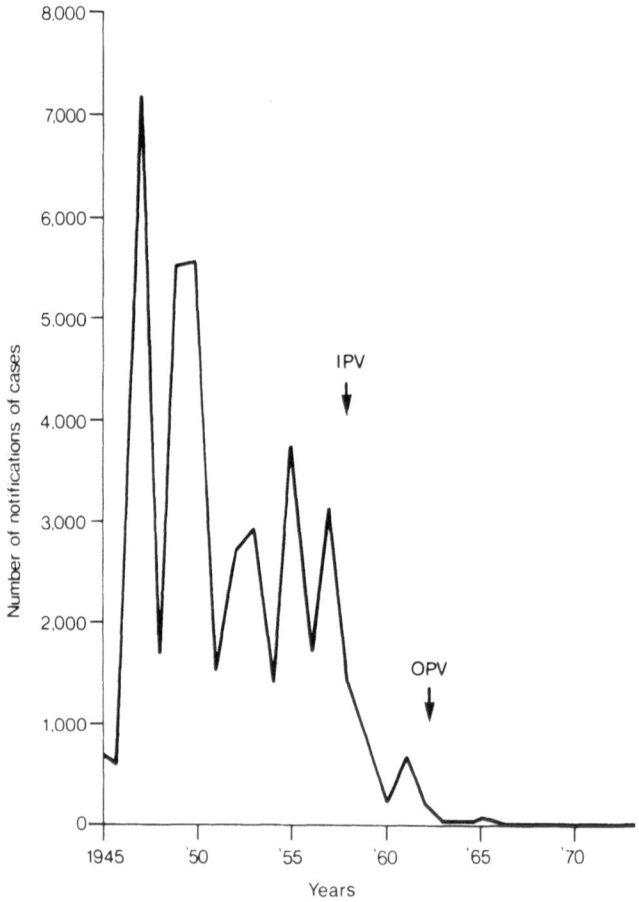

Figure 5   Notifications of paralytic poliomyelitis (England and Wales). IPV = inactivated poliovirus vaccine; OPV = oral poliovirus vaccine

of age. Until after World War II there were small scattered outbreaks in various parts of Britain but none of them was on the scale of the epidemics occurring at that time in Scandinavia or the USA. Then in 1947 there was a sudden increase in incidence and the total number of cases rose to 7776 compared with the previous highest figure of 1589 in 1938. During this century there has also been change in age of attack. Between 1912 (when the disease became notifiable) and 1920, about 65% of cases were in the 0–4-year-old group and 30% in the 5–14-year-olds. In contrast, between 1942 and 1950 one third of cases were in each of the 0–4, 5–14 and over-15 age groups.

Why there was a sudden increase in 1947 remains a mystery. Yearly epidemics of varying severity continued until 1958 when vaccine was introduced (Figure 5). After that, what Simon Flexner called 'this saddest of diseases', which left many persons permanently paralysed, appears to have become a thing of the past in North America and much of Europe and nowadays, in developed countries, poliomyelitis is a disease of the non-immunized.

The shift from endemic to epidemic poliomyelitis has followed this characteristic pattern in all countries, and it appears that the incidence of poliomyelitis bears an inverse relation to infant mortality. When the number of deaths per 1000 live births falls below 75, poliomyelitis changes from an endemic to an epidemic disease. The implication of these findings for developing countries is obvious.

## Natural history

Polioviruses enter the body by the mouth and replicate in the pharynx, the intestine and lymph nodes.

The virus may get into the blood (depending on the virus strain) and the viraemia which may occur in a number of individuals can lead to invasion of the c.n.s. with subsequent destruction of neurons leading to paralysis. However, paralysis is a rare outcome, and the vast majority of infections with polioviruses have always gone unrecognized. Depending on the strain of the virus and the susceptibility of population, there may be from about 100 to 1000 or more subclinical infections to each clinical case.

Of the three types of polioviruses, Type 1 has been responsible for about 60% of all paralytic cases in the northern hemisphere. Although there are minor antigenic similarities between the three types, all have similar characteristics and, with the exception of the Type 3 virus, the immunity to each of them is essentially type-specific.

The viruses are transmitted from person to person by the faecal-oral route, but no one knows if oropharyngeal virus or faecal virus is the more important in the spread of the disease.

## Vaccines

There are two types of poliovirus vaccines, namely inactivated poliovirus vaccines (IPV) and live attenuated oral poliovirus vaccines (OPV).

While only the latter is at present recommended for routine use in the UK, in the USA and in most other countries, it must not be forgotten that poliomyelitis was nearly completely controlled in the UK by IPV (Figure 5). It is still the only type of vaccine in routine use in Sweden and the Netherlands and until very recently in Finland, where OPV has been used temporarily prior to the introduction of more potent IPV. Some IPV is also used in Canada. Poliomyelitis has been eradicated from Sweden with IPV, and in the Netherlands the disease has occurred only rarely since the introduction of inactivated vaccines (essentially in communities which have resisted immunization on religious grounds).

In Finland the immunization programme was based on the use of six doses of IPV with a coverage of over 90%. No cases of poliomyelitis had been reported during the two decades prior to 1984 when seven cases of poliomyelitis due to a 'wild' Type 3 virus were found and the virus seemed to be fairly widely distributed. Serological surveys prior to this outbreak had shown that in children aged 1–6 years antibody to Type 3 virus was detectable in only 47–60% of them, but in 62–67% and 83–93% to Types 1 and 2 respectively. While this outbreak is somewhat surprising it would appear to be due to low antigenicity of the components of the vaccine, but at the same time there is some evidence that the Type 3 virus strain isolated was poorly neutralized by antibodies to the classical vaccine strain of Type 3 virus, suggesting that some antigenic evolution has occurred in this virus.

## Inactivated poliovirus vaccines (IPV)

These are manufactured by growing each type of poliovirus in tissue culture and inactivating the virus-rich tissue culture fluids with formalin. The fluids are then filtered and tested for purity and their antigenicity is measured and expressed in D units. The three types of inactivated viruses are then blended in the required proportions. Most vaccines nowadays contain in the region of 40 D Antigenic Units (DAU) for poliovirus Type 1, 8 for Type 2 and 32 for Type 3 per dose.

When potent vaccines are used and given at properly spaced intervals, IPV stimulates high levels of neutralizing antibody. As with other inactivated antigens, primary immunization with IPV sensitizes the body to react with a secondary response when the antigen is encountered again, either as an infection or when the individual is given a booster injection of vaccine. Salk is of the opinion that a state of durable immunity to paralytic polio is more closely correlated with the presence of immunological memory than with detectable levels of serum antibody, and that such immunity can be induced by a single dose of potent IPV.

The immunity induced by IPV is essentially due to circulating antibodies which neutralize the virus and prevent its spread from the alimentary canal to the c.n.s. The levels of antibody which can be attained by IPV are higher than those induced by OPV and it seems that this serological immunity is as durable as that following OPV, if not more so. In one survey in the UK done some years ago, in comparing the responses in children to previous immunization with IPV and OPV it was found that the antibody levels stimulated by potent IPV approximate the maximum obtainable, and are subsequently more readily boosted by a single injection of IPV than by a dose of OPV.

## Herd immunity

It is not always appreciated that IPV has a profound epidemiological effect in preventing the spread of polioviruses. As noted above, in Sweden where only IPV had been used routinely, both poliomyelitis and polioviruses have disappeared.

It has been shown that when live poliovirus is given to individuals immunized with IPV, not only can virus not be recovered from the oropharynx, but also faecal excretion of virus is greatly reduced, to a level which makes it unlikely that such immunized persons would transmit the disease if they were infected.

## *Evidence of protection*

Following the field trials of IPV in the USA in 1954/1955 and the early trials in the UK, it was seen that even without complete vaccine coverage of the susceptible populations this vaccine was capable of producing a tenfold reduction in paralytic attack rates during the next 5 years. While IPV produced a dramatic effect on the incidence of paralytic poliomyelitis in Europe and in North America, there was a small rise in the incidence and deaths from poliomyelitis in 1960 and 1961 (Figures 5 and 6).

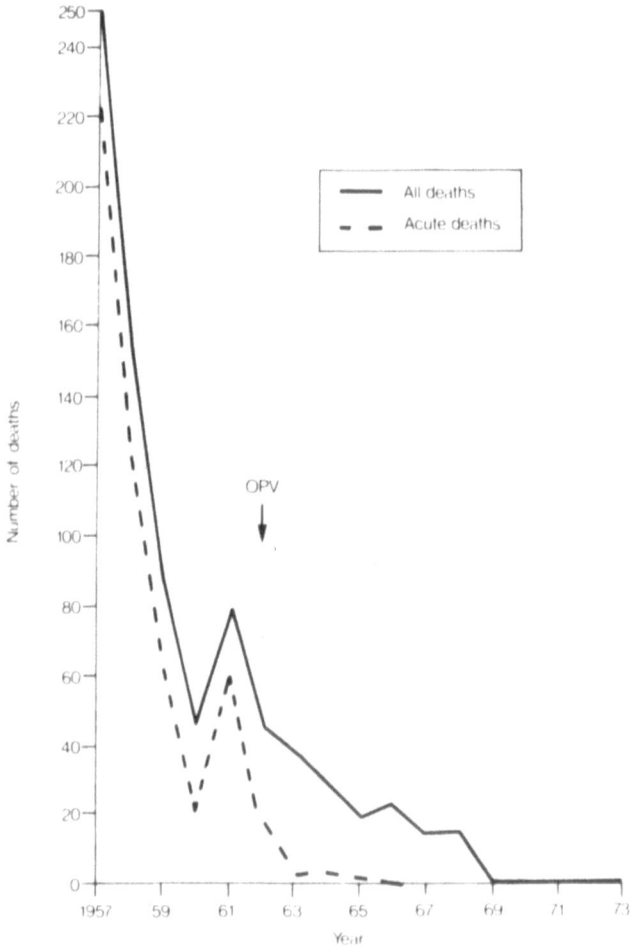

**Figure 6**   Deaths from poliomyelitis, 1957–73 (England and Wales)

This rise was explained by the relatively poor antigenicity of the Type 1 component of the vaccine. In early vaccines this was the least effective antigen, though Type 1 virus was the most frequently paralytic virus.

Because of the high efficacy of the Type 2 component in the vaccine, Type 2 virus practically disappeared from those countries with effective immunization programmes. However, no effort was made to improve IPV at that time, for it was generally considered that a better vaccine (OPV) was just around the corner. Nevertheless, with a relatively impotent IPV, poliomyelitis was almost eliminated from countries with good immunization programmes. The potency of the IPV which is available today is at least ten times greater than that of vaccines produced in the late 1950s. The continued efficacy of IPV in countries which have used only IPV for routine immunization is clearly established. It is important to realize that it is relatively simple to change the composition of IPV without extensive field trials. This is not possible with OPV. There are, however, still some questions to be answered in relation to the best age for immunization and the number of doses required, particularly in developing countries (see Chapter 12).

## Reactions

In the early days of IPV it was found that live virus was present in some batches of vaccine which produced paralytic poliomyelitis in some inoculated children and their contacts. However, since 1962, with improved manufacturing and safety-testing techniques, IPV has been one of the safest vaccines available.

Side-effects are rare: some IPV contains traces of streptomycin and neomycin and the possibility of reactions in sensitive individuals must be remembered. In general, with millions of doses, only a few complications like the Guillain–Barré syndrome, encephalopathy and convulsions have been recorded. All of these could have occurred by chance and be unassociated with the immunization. Since purified vaccines were introduced, adverse effects seem to have been even less frequent.

## Special use of IPV

IPV is the vaccine of choice for non-immunized adults, because the risk of vaccine-associated paralysis following OPV is slightly higher in adults than in children.

Dip/tet/polio, if available, is preferable to dip/tet and OPV at school entry for, as noted, IPV more regularly boosts circulating antibody than does a single dose of OPV.

Where IPV is not used routinely it should be made available for individuals in whom OPV is contraindicated - which includes pregnant women, patients undergoing corticosteroid therapy or those with intestinal dysfunction. Although OPV is usually contraindicated for pregnant women there is no evidence that a pregnant woman infected with poliovirus will transmit it to her fetus. If her baby does become infected, this would appear to occur during childbirth.

### Quadruple vaccine

A quadruple dip/tet/pert/IPV vaccine was extensively tested in N. Ireland in the 1960s and began to be routinely used in that province and in parts of England but was disappointingly withdrawn because of the reactions to the pertussis component available at that time. It is worth noting that all the laboratory controlled studies f this vaccine were made in babies over 6 months of age and it was not until it was given routinely in younger babies that reactions to the pertussis component became apparent (pages 11, 44). At the same time a successful quadruple vaccine was developed in Canada and has been in use in various parts of that country for many years (Table 12).

**Table 12** Recommended schedule for infants and children, using quadruple vaccine, as in Canada

| Age | Immunization |
| --- | --- |
| 2 months | Dip/pert/tet/polio (quad) |
| 4 months | Dip/pert/tet/polio (quad) |
| 6 months | Dip/pert/tet/polio (quad) |
| 1 y | Measles vaccine |
| | Rubella vaccine* |
| 1½ y | Dip/pert/tet/polio (quad) |
| 4–6 y | Dip/pert/tet/polio (quad) |
| 11–12 y (females only) | Rubella vaccine* |
| 14–16 y | Dip/tet/polio |

* At or after 1 year to infants of both sexes or at 12 years to prepubertal girls

In recent years an antigenically improved quadruple vaccine has been developed at the Rijks Institute in the Netherlands which contains dip (15 Lf)/tet (10 Lf)/pert (16 OU*) and polio type 1, 2 and 3 with 40, 8 and 32 D-antigen units respectively. This vaccine has been subjected to several field trials and it has been found that the serological responses have been excellent. The results of epidemiological surveillance look promising and are awaited with interest. Studies are also being made with two-dose schedules of this vaccine. The evidence that all the components of this vaccine will be equally effective in producing adequate protection after two suitably spaced doses is encouraging.

## Oral poliovaccine

This vaccine consists of attenuated strains of each of the three types of poliovirus (grown in tissue cultures) which have been selected for their lack of neurovirulence when the viruses are injected intraspinally or intracerebrally into monkeys. The vaccine virus fluids must be stringently tested in monkeys to confirm that they have maintained their avirulence and also in several systems to ensure that there are no extraneous contaminating agents present. These problems may be circumvented by using defined human diploid cell lines for virus culture.

Types 1, 2 and 3 attenuated strains may be given separately as monovalent vaccines, but for administrative convenience all three types of vaccine are usually given together as a trivalent preparation. The number of virus particles contained in a single dose of trivalent vaccine is usually about $10^6$ for Type 1, $10^5$ for Type 2 and $10^{5.5}$ for Type 3. (In the UK this vaccine is now available in single dose ampoules.)

### Action of OPV

OPV viruses, like wild polioviruses, multiply in the throat and in the intestine. They stimulate not only circulating antibodies (IgM and IgG) but also IgA which prevents infection of the intestinal canal.

The immunity with OPV is dependent on replication of the viruses in the gut: if the vaccine viruses do not multiply the individual will not become immunized. If the vaccine is given to an individual who, for

---

* Opacity units

example, is immune to Type 2 virus as a result of previous immunization or a previous natural Type 2 infection, the Type 2 vaccine virus would not replicate. However, one or both of the other types could infect and immunize.

One virus can interfere with the replication of another. When trivalent vaccine is fed, only one of the virus types will colonize the gut and multiply to begin with and stimulate immunity to that type. One of the other types in the vaccine may remain in the gut and take over when the first colonizing type has ceased to replicate, and so immunity to two types could follow a dose of trivalent OPV. (On the other hand immunity to a second type may not develop till the second dose, while immunity to two types *could* follow a second dose.) I have no experience of a successful 'take' of all three types following a single dose of trivalent vaccine. All sorts of combinations of success or failure to immunize against any one type can occur when oral vaccines are given, for other entero viruses can interfere with polioviruses. Thus, if a child is carrying an entero virus, e.g. an ECHO or Coxsackie virus – many of which give subclinical infections – then again there may be interference with the vaccine 'take' when OPV is given.

## Schedule of immunization

OPV does not readily colonize the guts of small babies. It is usually given at the same time as dip/tet/pert, i.e. the first dose at 3–6 months of age, the second 6 weeks later and the third 6 months later. A reinforcing dose should be given at school entry and another one at school leaving.

In addition to routine immunization of babies (see schedule, Chapter 2) attention should be paid to immunizing young adults who may have escaped immunization in childhood and consider themselves too old for immunization. With the disappearance of wild viruses, they could possibly also have escaped a natural immunizing infection, but IPV is preferable for immunization of adults.

## Safety of OPV

Live virus vaccines carry more potential hazards than inactivated ones. In the first place, the tissue culture passages of the OPV virus may lead to an increase in its neurovirulence compared with the seed virus from which it originated. This has been a recurring problem in the manufacture of OPV, which requires the meticulous testing of neurovirulence of the virus pool in monkeys and the comparison of the level of neurovirulence with that of reference strains. Secondly, a whole battery of tests is required to ensure that there is no contamination of the vaccine virus with extraneous agents. Thirdly, there is the problem that occasionally the attenuated vaccine virus becomes less attenuated on replication in the human gut. Although this danger is much less than had been anticipated, it must be kept in mind not only as a risk to persons vaccinated but also to their contacts. These problems do not arise with IPV.

The overall risk of paralytic poliomyelitis associated with OPV in persons vaccinated and their contacts is of the order of one to three per million doses but this figure relates to communities with a variable proportion of naturally immune individuals. The exact risk in a susceptible population is unknown: it appears to be greater with Type 2 and Type 3 than with Type 1 vaccine virus.

Because of the possible risk to contacts, when vaccine is being given to the baby of young parents it is important that they should be offered vaccine at the same time, for parents have been paralysed from the progeny of vaccine virus from their own babies. Also, babies who have recently received vaccine should not be put in contact with non-immunized infants. (There is presumptive evidence that one who had been put in a pram with a recently vaccinated baby contracted a paralytic infection.)

Since the introduction of poliovirus vaccines the UK Public Health Laboratory Service and the CDC (now the Infectious Disease Center) in Atlanta, Georgia, have carried out surveillance of all cases of poliomyelitis. Vaccine viruses have certain growth characteristics in the laboratory and it was often possible to identify viruses as having the properties of 'wild virus' or of a 'vaccine virus'. In the UK, of 163 strains isolated in 1972, only ten had the characteristics of 'wild' viruses, In the past, it was difficult to characterize strains serologically in order to decide whether or not a strain recovered from a paralytic or non-paralytic case was or was not vaccine-derived, for very occasionally vaccine viruses may develop the paralytic properties of 'wild' strains and while some appear to retain the serological markers of the vaccine virus, others may lose them and appear to be 'wild' viruses. Recent work using strain-specific absorbed sera and oligonucleotide mapping (fingerprinting) techniques has greatly facilitated epidemiological studies and the identification of the origin of viruses from paralytic and non-paralytic cases.

## Efficacy of OPV

Paralytic and non-paralytic poliomyelitis has virtually disappeared from all countries where there has been good coverage with OPV (as with potent IPV). Now that poliomyelitis is rarely found in the UK and USA, is it necessary to continue to immunize against it? The answer is an emphatic YES, for there is still much poliomyelitis throughout the world. While it has tended to disappear from countries with effective immunization programmes, notifications have increased in some less fortunate developing countries. Poliovirus can be imported 'silently' from many parts of the world and could spread readily in a poorly immunized community. Failure to maintain effective immunization programmes in developed countries could lead to a return to an epidemic situation.

It is important to realize that a 75% immunization rate in children is not enough. We should be attempting to achieve near 100% acceptance rates for both primary immunizations and for boosters at school entry and school leaving.

## Special cases: international travel and immigrants

Travellers from countries where poliomyelitis has been controlled going to countries where it is endemic or epidemic should appreciate that they are at increased risk and should be fully immunized. Those who have been immunized as infants or children with OPV should be given a booster of IPV. Those who have not been immunized or who have only completed part of a course should complete the course and have an additional reinforcing dose of vaccine. IPV is preferred for unvaccinated adults, but where there is an urgent need for immunization prior to travel a single dose of trivalent OPV is probably the most effective measure. (*See also* Chapter 11.)

Particular attention should be given to immunizing immigrant families who may have come from countries with no routine poliomyelitis immunization programme. Indeed at the present time in several European countries the majority of the cases of poliomyelitis in children involve the families of migrant workers from endemic areas.

## Outbreak control

Presumably the interference effect of OPV comes into play before the development of protective levels of neutralizing antibody. This interference phenomenon can be used to control an outbreak. Thus, if a case of poliomyelitis occurs, all contacts, e.g. in school, play area and street, should immediately be given a dose of OPV, regardless of their previous history of immunization. The efficacy of this 'fire brigade' action will depend on local conditions but it should limit the spread of wild strains because of interference induced by the attenuated vaccine viruses.

How interference works is not certain, but presumably the attenuated vaccine virus colonizes the gut and prevents the epidemic strain from attaching to cell receptors.

In the USA, poliomyelitis is considered to be epidemic (or potentially epidemic) when there are two or more cases caused by the same type of virus during a 4-week period in a defined population. Under these circumstances all persons 6 weeks of age or older who have not previously been immunized are offered a complete course of OPV.

## Surveillance

Efficacy must be continuously monitored. Recent studies in places as far apart as Glasgow and Ivanjua in Serbia (where immunization programmes have been carried out with OPV) have indicated gaps in immunity in school children and young adults. These studies do not support the belief that attenuated strains of OPV will necessarily give lifelong immunity. It may be that vaccine strains are less antigenic than 'wild' ones or that repeated experiences with vaccine-type viruses may be necessary to maintain immunity now that boosting effect of 'wild' strains has virtually disappeared from some countries. Booster doses of vaccine in addition to those given at school entry and school leaving may come to be required.

## Adverse reactions

The only adverse reaction is the very slight risk of paralytic polio-myelitis induced by OPV.

## Contraindications

The contraindications to OPV are similar to those of other live viruses. While OPV should not be given to anyone with an acute illness including diarrhoea or other acute or severe intestinal dysfunction, minor illnesses such as colds and coughs are not considered to be contraindications.

The vaccine should not be given to severe hypogammaglobu-linaemia subjects, for they appear more liable to develop paralysis after exposure to both vaccine and 'wild' strains. Moreover, they may become prolonged carriers of virus in high titre in their gastro-intestinal tracts. OPV should not be given to patients on corti-costeroids or immunosuppressive therapy. All in this group of individuals may be immunized with IPV.

## Storage of OPV

OPV is stored in bulk at $-20\,°C$ and remains viable for at least 6 months. After issue from the deep freeze, like all other vaccines it should be held at about $+4\,°C$.

## Past and future

Most doctors now entering general practice may never see a case of paralytic poliomyelitis, but many of them were schoolchildren in the year when 7000 or more paralytic cases were notified in England and Wales alone, of whom more than 700 died. Truly, poliovaccine has been a success story. The stability of the neurovirulence of polioviruses presents a continuous problem and must be carefully monitored, both in the community and in the production of vaccines. Surveillance of the immunity status of the population is of high priority.

About a quarter of a century ago, my colleagues and I published the results of a satisfactory small scale laboratory controlled clinical trial of a quintuple vaccine consisting of dip/tet/pertussis/IPV and measles (haemagglutinin) and there is no reason why this type of vaccine and indeed a sextuple inactivated vaccine with a rubella component should not be developed. Other antigens could also be added. This is the way in which I think that immunization will go in the future, made possible by the recent developments in tissue culture techniques, in recombinant DNA technology and molecular genetics. Antigens for vaccines could be weighted out and mixed to give predictable antibody levels and durable immunity.

# 7
# Measles (Rubeola)

Measles is caused by a virus belonging to the myxovirus group and it can be prevented by immunization, which has virtually eradicated the disease from some countries.

## The virus

The virus is a RNA containing paramyxovirus and there is only one serological type. Man is the only natural host although the virus may be transmitted to monkeys and apes. It can be grown in chick embryos and in tissue cultures of chick-embryo fibroblasts and in human and monkey-cell cultures in which it produces multinucleated syncytial giant cells. The virus has several antigens including haemagglutinins which stimulate protective antibodies which may be measured by neutralization, haemagglutination inhibition and complement fixation tests.

## The disease

The disease is characterized by fever and catarrhal symptoms followed in 3–4 days by a red, blotchy rash. Koplik spots may be present on the buccal mucosa before or after the onset of the rash. In developed countries, some have considered that measles seems to have become a relatively benign disease in recent years. However, in the UK there is still an average of 100 000 cases a year with about 20 deaths. Postal surveys in the UK have indicated that chest complications and otitis media occur in about 3% or 4% of infections and 'neurological illness' in about four per 1000 cases. The exact definition of 'neurological illness' has been unsatisfactory in these studies, but it seems that about 1:1000 to 1:10 000 children with measles showed some impaired consciousness or evidence of encephalitis. The true incidence of neurological complications associated with measles infection is probably more in the region of 1:10 000, but varies with time and place.

Rare complications include post-infectious encephalomyelitis and subacute sclerosing panencephalitis*. In the UK the hospital admission rate for cases of measles is about 1%. The case fatality rate is 0.2/1000 in most developed countries but 400 or 500 times greater in parts of the Third World.

## Natural history

Susceptibility to measles is universal and the disease is nearly always a clinical one. Before the introduction of vaccine nearly all children had had an attack of measles before puberty and this provided a lifelong immunity to measles in almost everyone. The total number of cases in any country without an immunization programme should therefore be approximately the same as the number of births. Obviously, there was and is much undernotification.

By the middle of the 18th century outbreaks of measles in London began to show a biennial periodicity as sufficient susceptibles accumulated to provide a critical number to initiate an epidemic, and with the decline in smallpox in the early part of the 19th century measles became a more prominent disease, as evidenced by mortality figures.

Between 1900 and 1950 the death rate from measles in the UK fell from about 300 to 2.0 per million population. This was in part related to smaller family size, better social conditions and medical care. It is not surprising that the Decennial Supplement of the Registrar General for 1931 for England and Wales showed that the mortality from measles of children aged 1 year in what was social class V was about 20 times greater than those in social class I.

## Notifications

The notification of measles was introduced in late 1939. The introduction of antibiotics in the latter years of the 40s may have had a slight influence on the case fatality rates (Table 13).

---

* A disease which occurs at 7-10 years in previously healthy children who have been infected with measles virus when young and in whom the virus awakes from a latent state in the c.n.s.

MEASLES (RUBEOLA)

**Table 13**  Notifications of measles

| Year | 1945 | 1946 | 1947 | 1948 | 1949 | 1950 | 1951 | 1952 | 1953 | 1954 | 1955 |
|---|---|---|---|---|---|---|---|---|---|---|---|
| Notifications: 1000s | 446.8 | 160.4 | 393.8 | 399.6 | 385.9 | 367.7 | 616.2 | 389.5 | 545.0 | 147.0 | 693.8 |
| Fatality ratio per 10 000 notifications | 16 | 13 | 16 | 8 | 8 | 6 | 5 | 4 | 4 | 3 | 2 |

**Table 14**  Notifications and deaths England and Wales from 1958 when comparable data available (Annual Reports CMO)

| Year | Notifications | Deaths | Fatality ratio per 100 notifications |
|---|---|---|---|
| 1958 | 259 398 | 49 | 0.02 |
| 59 | 539 524 | 98 | 0.02 |
| 1960 | 159 364 | 31 | 0.02 |
| 61 | 763 531 | 152 | 0.02 |
| 62 | 184 895 | 39 | 0.02 |
| 63 | 601 255 | 127 | 0.02 |
| 64 | 306 801 | 73 | 0.02 |
| 65 | 502 209 | 115 | 0.02 |
| 66 | 343 642 | 80 | 0.02 |
| 67 | 460 407 | 99 | 0.02 |
| 68* | 236 154 | 51 | 0.02 |
| 69 | 142 111 | 36 | 0.03 |
| 1970 | 307 408 | 42 | 0.01 |
| 71 | 135 241 | 28 | 0.02 |
| 72 | 145 916 | 29 | 0.02 |
| 73 | 152 578 | 33 | 0.02 |
| 74 | 109 636 | 20 | 0.02 |
| 75 | 143 072 | 16 | 0.01 |
| 76 | 55 502 | 14 | 0.03 |
| 77 | 173 361 | 23 | 0.01 |
| 78 | 124 067 | 20 | 0.02 |
| 79 | 77 363 | 17 | 0.02 |
| 1980 | 139 487 | 26 | 0.02 |
| 81 | 52 979 | 15 | 0.02 |
| 82 | 94 195 | 13 | 0.01 |
| 83 | 103 700 | 16 | 0.01 |
| 84 | 62 079 | 10 | 0.01 |
| 85 | — | — | — |

* Introduction of measles vaccines

69

The notifications, deaths and case fatality rates from 1958 to 1984 are shown in Table 14. Between 1974 and 1983 there has been an average of about 19 deaths each year from measles in the UK, and about half of these occurred in children with some serious disability or chronic disease. It is surprising how little change there has been till very recently in the case fatality rates over the years.

In developed countries prior to the introduction of vaccine, the incidence of measles was highest in the 3–5-years age group, in contrast to places such as Nigeria where 50% of children become infected by 2 years of age and 75% by 3 years of age.

The mortality in some developing countries today is similar to what it was in England and Wales at the beginning of this century.

## Measles vaccines

### Live measles virus vaccines

The earliest attempts to vaccinate against measles were made in Edinburgh in 1758 by Dr Francis Home, who tried to modify the disease by the inoculation of blood from a patient. (This method was presumably influenced by variolation for the prevention of smallpox – see page 188.) However, it was not until the virus was adapted to grow in tissue cultures that the preparation of vaccines became practicable, and their development followed rapidly on that of poliomyelitis vaccine. The techniques for manufacturing were similar, and the criteria for the acceptability of live virus vaccines, as far as safety and immunogenicity were concerned, had already been worked out from experience with poliovirus vaccines. Indeed, in some respects it had become easier to make virus vaccines than to have them accepted by the medical profession and by parents.

### Killed measles virus vaccine

Early experiments with killed measles vaccine (KMV) looked very hopeful. A course of three injections of formalin-inactivated virus gave up to 95% antibody conversion rates. Furthermore, there were none of the symptoms of mild infections with measles which followed the use of live attenuated strains. Unfortunately, when some children who had been immunized with KMV were challenged with live measles virus vaccine (LMV) they often developed what appeared to be an Arthus type of reaction with pain, erythema and induration at the site of inoculation. Some immunized children exposed to natural infections developed very odd and sometimes severe respiratory conditions, urticaria and petechial and purpuric reactions. The reasons for this are uncertain, but it would seem that after immunization with the KMV available at that time, the original levels of neutralizing antibody fell rapidly but the individuals remained hypersensitive.

Another type of purified and inactivated vaccine was prepared from the haemagglutinin fraction of measles virus. Studies done with this type of measles vaccine included a small trial of dip/tet/pert/polio/measles vaccine (see page 66) containing a measles haemagglutinin component. The seroconversion rates were good and no reactions occurred in the vaccinees when they were subsequently challenged with live virus, but the numbers tested were very small.

## Live measles virus vaccine

The earliest experimental live measles vaccine was prepared from a strain of virus derived from a patient (called Edmonston) which became attenuated by being passed through human and chick-embryo tissue cultures. This attenuated strain produced about a 95% antibody conversion rate but also produced fever, rash, upper respiratory symptoms and sometimes convulsions in a high proportion of immunized children. The 'vaccine disease', although non-communicable, was too like the natural infection. Attempts were made to modify these vaccine reactions by giving an injection of pooled immunoglobulin at the same time as the vaccine, but this was hardly an acceptable procedure.

Attempts were also made to precede the injection of the attenuated virus vaccine by actively immunizing with killed measles vaccine (see above) but, as noted, this procedure produced some untoward results. Accordingly, attempts were made to develop further attenuated strains. The most satisfactory vaccine virus was developed from the Schwarz strain. This was a chick-embryo tissue culture (CETC) strain derived from the Edmonston B strain by repeated passages in CETC at low temperature. This vaccine produced fewer reactions but a seroconversion rate somewhat lower than that of more virulent vaccine viruses. This vaccine virus is not transmitted from those vaccinated to contacts.

## Immunization

The vaccine is provided as a freeze dried live virus preparation with diluent for reconstitution and sterile disposable syringes and needles. It is given by deep subcutaneous or intramuscular injection.

## Routine schedule of immunization

It is recommended that measles vaccine should be given routinely in the second year of life, because the presence of maternal antibody which persists up to about 9 months of age may inhibit the replication of the vaccine virus and the subsequent development of antibodies.

In some places there are considerable advantages in postponing immunization until about 3 years of age (see below, Reactions), but in any event every effort must be made to try to ensure that every child entering nursery school or primary school has been immunized. This is a legal requirement in the USA at the present time, in that no child may enter school unless he or she has been immunized against measles (and other common infectious diseases). As a result of this policy it appears that measles has ceased to be transmitted in the USA except from importations from foreign countries.

In areas where there is a high probability of infection at an early age, the vaccine has been given to infants as early as 6 months of age. This procedure is of doubtful value because of the variable sero-conversion rate in children under 1 year of age: if this is done, a second dose of vaccine must be given at 9-12 months of age.

In addition to routine immunization in the second year of life, it is important to ensure that all susceptible entrants to nursery and primary school are immunized; vaccine should be offered to any older children who have not had a clinical attack of measles. There is no age bar.

Although the clinical diagnosis of measles is easy, an assertion that an individual has had measles should not be accepted as a reason for not carrying out routine immunization unless the attack of measles is confirmed by a medical attendant. No harm will come of giving vaccine to a child who has actually had measles.

For *combined measles/mumps/rubella* (MMR) vaccine, see page 90.

## Effectiveness

From field studies it appears that the overall protection rate* is in the region of 85%. Vaccine induced antibody appears to be durable up to 16 years of age in the UK where, of course, 'wild' virus is still circulating; but it seems reasonable to assume at present that protection will be durable. Waning immunity could be important where 'wild' viruses have ceased to circulate.

The effect of immunization on notifications has been directly related to the vaccine coverage. After the introduction of vaccine in 1968 in the UK there was a drop in the number of notifications and deaths (see Table 14) but, unlike the achievements made with diphtheria and poliomyelitis vaccines, the eradication of measles in the UK seems a long way off. There is no use in hoping that when 75% of the susceptible population has been immunized, measles in the UK, like diphtheria, will no longer be transmitted in the community. Measles epidemics have continued to occur in some communities with 75% or higher rates of immunization. These epidemics are separated by longer intervals and have tended to involve older age groups than before immunization. In some places where immunization programmes have been introduced, measles seems to have become a low grade endemic infection.

It has been pointed out from a study of Bartlett's epidemiological model that in the UK there is a critical community size of the order of a quarter of a million above which measles can maintain itself more or less indefinitely in the population. In a population of that size there will be a sufficient number of susceptibles from those not infected in previous epidemics and from those migrating into or being born in the areas. With populations less than a quarter of a million, measles could die out after an epidemic, and it would not recur unless reintroduced (as in the classical outbreak described by Dr Panum in 1846 in the Faeroe Islands).

After a partial vaccination programme with an 85% effective vaccine, it has been predicted that the interval between measles epidemics will increase. Furthermore, relative to the size of the

---

* Protection rates are calculated as:

$$\frac{\text{Attack rate in unvaccinated} - \text{Attack rate in vaccinated}}{\text{Attack rate in unvaccinated}} \times 100$$

susceptible population, epidemics will be larger after vaccination than before (although smaller in absolute numbers). The previous biennial cycle may become a 3-4-year cycle and the age at attack will increase. As far as the critical community size is concerned, this would increase as the immunization rates increase. However, a vaccine acceptance rate of perhaps 100% (with a 90% effective vaccine) might be required to increase the critical community size above the total population in a homogeneous community. With the lack of homogeneity of the population a lower rate would presumably be adequate. Even so, the possibility of reintroduction will be present for years to come, and to prevent outbreaks of measles after importations a very high level of immunization will have to be maintained.

In the UK, with very incomplete vaccine coverage, measles is still essentially a disease of the 1-4 age group, and there has been no apparent rise in age incidence. Although there has been a marked reduction in the incidence of measles in children, the proportion of cases in older age groups has not been falling. It is as yet uncertain how important are 'boosts' with 'wild' virus in maintaining life-long immunity, but those countries which have achieved eradication of measles virus may in the future be faced with problems of re-emergence of the disease.

In the USA, with high vaccine coverage in children, outbreaks of measles have been occurring among students who had escaped child-hood immunization by vaccine or natural infections following the decrease in circulation of 'wild virus', and at the present time in the USA, measles in college students accounts for a substantial proportion of morbidity and in an outbreak on one campus there was a case fatality over 2%. The susceptibility of college students in the USA has been said to be about 15%, which makes colleges a potential site for sustained outbreaks. In view, of this, proof of measles immunization is being required before matriculation; this will involve the whole population of students who were babies about the mid-1960s before routine immunization. Since measles is nearly always a clinically recognized disease it should be possible to screen the few potentially susceptible individuals for the absence of measles antibody.

Now that measles vaccine has been recommended for routine use we must encourage its use for all children who have not had a natural infection. Otherwise, as measles becomes controlled, they will grow up having had no contact with wild measles virus and a natural infection incurred as an adolescent or an adult may be more of a nuisance and more severe than an infection in childhood. Furthermore, it is said that the incidence of measles encephalitis in children over 10 years of age is 'considerably higher' than in younger children.

## Outbreak control

When cases occur in countries with well developed immunization programmes and good vaccine coverage, it would seem sensible to invoke the 'fire brigade' technique in that immediate steps should be taken to immunize home, school, playmate and other susceptible children within 72 hours of contact with a case. As with poliomyelitis control, the extent of the operation will depend on local conditions. Routine immunization programmes should not be disrupted by what may be an expensive and sometimes futile outbreak control. It is only of value in well immunized communities and the vaccine will only be effective if given within 72 hours of contact with a case. During an outbreak, human normal immunoglobulin should be given to all children for whom vaccine is contraindicated and who are at special risk. The recommended dose is: under 1 year – 0.25 g; 1–2 years – 0.5 g; over 3 years – 0.75 g (see Chapter 13).

## Reactions

The available vaccine produces a number of reactions. These are most marked in infants and diminish up to 3 or 4 years of age which, as already mentioned, may be a more suitable age to offer vaccine.

About 7–10 days after immunization most children have some malaise and about one third of them have a transient rash and a mild febrile reaction. Febrile convulsions may be associated with any febrile condition in children. These are most frequent in the 1-year and 2-year age groups (eight per 1000) falling in the 3-year-olds to about six per 1000 and rapidly dropping in older children. So it could be that any child who develops fever after measles vaccine might have a convulsion. It is of course possible that vaccine may be given to a child who is incubating some infection and that the convulsion is not related to the vaccine but to the concurrent infection. A convulsion may follow any immunization by chance and it is not easy to collect accurate data on the association of convulsions with measles vaccine, but the probability of a convulsion following infection with measles is probably about ten times greater than after immunization with measles vaccine.

## Encephalitis

Some of the very early batches of vaccine which were on the market about 20 years ago were associated with a few cases of encephalitis and the memory of this still lingers on. Nowadays, this is an exceedingly rare vaccine complication. It was suggested that the incidence of encephalitis during the acute stage of measles (acute encephalitis) or with onset about 10 days later (acute post-infectious encephalomyelitis) is probably about 1:1000 to 1:10000; the occurrence of 'encephalitis' after immunization is probably of the order of less than 1:100000. This is merely an estimate, for there is no clear guidance for the diagnosis of encephalitis. I think that it can be safely assumed that the vaccine has prevented ten times more natural cases of encephalitis than it is likely to have caused.

## Subacute sclerosing panencephalitis (SSPE)

The risk of SSPE (a latent infection of the brain with measles virus) following vaccination with live virus measles vaccine appears to be about one tenth of the risk associated with 'wild' measles virus. Indeed with the drop in the incidence of measles in countries with immunization programmes, SSPE is apparently becoming even more rare than in the past. Measles vaccine significantly reduces the chance of developing SSPE.

## Other reactions

An anaphylactic reaction to measles vaccine might occur as with any other vaccine so, as always, adrenaline should be to hand as a precaution. A nephrotic syndrome after measles vaccination has been reported. Any such case should be discussed with an immunologist so that they can be immediately investigated.

## Contraindications

Routine measles vaccination is absolutely contraindicated in individuals suffering from conditions where live virus vaccines are contraindicated, i.e. leukaemia, Hodgkin's disease, or other diseases of the lymphoid or mononuclear phagocytic system (reticuloendothelial system). Children with deficiencies of immune mechanisms or undergoing corticosteroid or immunosuppressive therapy should not be vaccinated, but discussions with a paediatrician or other specialist of the disease in question should take place to decide what modification of the routine immunization procedure might be made to protect them for they will be more liable to a serious outcome if they develop measles.

Measles vaccine is contraindicated in a child suffering from an acute febrile illness, and immunization should be postponed. If the child is recovering from an illness and has no fever, immunization is not contraindicated even if the child is still receiving antibiotics.

## Febrile convulsions

Children with a history of febrile convulsions, or whose parents or siblings have a history of convulsions (diagnosed as such by their medical attendant and 'not by granny') should be immunized under cover of a small quantity of immunoglobulin which is usually available from a local virus laboratory. The dose is usually 0.6 mg/lb body weight (0.04 ml/kg body weight in the USA, p. 00). This should be injected at the same time as the vaccine in a separate syringe in the opposite arm. The child becomes immunized under the passive protection of the measles antibodies present in normal immunoglobulin.

## Non-febrile convulsions

Careful consideration should be given to the immunization of children with a history of repeated non-febrile convulsions. It is preferable that immunization should be delayed until they are 3 years of age and a paediatrician should be consulted, who may then recommend that the immunization should be followed by an adequate course of an anticonvulsant.

## Antibiotics

Measles vaccine is contraindicated in persons hypersensitive to polymyxin or neomycin and to these antibiotics only.

## Not contraindications

### Sensitivity to eggs

Egg sensitivity is not a contraindication unless it is of an extreme anaphylactoid type. The vaccine virus is grown in chick fibroblasts which do not contain the allergens which are present in eggs. Similarly sensitivity to feathers is not a contraindication.

Allergies, asthma, hayfever, eczema, urticaria are not contraindications.

## Some special situations

### Special care units etc

Immunization is particularly important in special care units and other establishments for the care of normal or of handicapped children.

### Chronic diseases in children

Heart and lung diseases and other chronic diseases in children require special consideration for they are highly susceptible to serious infection with measles virus. Where there are contraindications, adverse reactions may be reduced by the use of immunoglobulin injected at the same time (see above).

### Pregnant women

While, as noted, live virus vaccines are not generally recommended for pregnant women, there is no evidence that measles vaccines may not be given safely and effectively to susceptible pregnant women who have been exposed to measles; however, on theoretical grounds it may be wiser to passively immunize them with normal immunoglobulin.

### Tuberculosis

Cell mediated and not humoral immunity seems to be the most important mechanism responsible for overcoming infections with measles or with tuberculosis. Measles virus inhibits the cell mediated response to tuberculin and individuals may become tuberculin negative for up to a month after infection or immunization with measles virus. An exacerbation of tuberculosis might occur in an individual with tuberculosis who was infected with measles virus, and therefore individuals known to have active tuberculosis should be under treatment when vaccinated, but the value of measles vaccine far outweighs the theoretical hazard of potential exacerbation of unsuspected tuberculosis.

## Vaccine storage

The package of vaccine and diluent should be stored in the cool part of a refrigerator, about $+4\,^{\circ}$C. They should not be frozen as this is likely to crack the ampoule of diluent. They should not be kept in the door of a refrigerator, where considerable variations in temperature can occur. After the contents of the ampoule of diluent (water for injection) has been added, the vaccine should be used as soon as possible and certainly within 1 hour. (The reconstituted vaccine may vary in colour from straw to pink.)

# 8
# Rubella

Rubella or German measles is caused by a virus which has many of the epidemiological properties of, and clinical similarities to, the paramyxoviruses (measles, parainfluenza, respiratory syncytial virus etc), but it is classified as a rubivirus. It may be prevented by a live virus vaccine.

## The virus

Rubella virus can be propagated in many different types of cell cultures including monkey and rabbit kidney and human-cell lines. There is only one antigenic type of the virus and one attack of the disease usually confers lifelong immunity, but this does not appear to be absolute and reinfections may occur although they are seldom associated with a viraemia and a rash.

## The disease

It is generally accepted that the name German measles came to be used after its identification by German physicians as a disease which was different from other exanthemata; however, some consider that the term was used to indicate that the disease was 'germain' (Old French = 'closely akin') to measles.

*In children and in adolescents* rubella is a relatively unimportant disease and the constitutional symptoms are so trivial that the illness is often not suspected till the rash is seen. The rash which may be morbilliform or scarlatiniform usually starts on the face and spreads rapidly over the trunk and limbs; it may be very fleeting, or obvious for only 1 or 2 days. Suboccipital and postauricular lymphadenopathy is frequent. In about 20% of infected adolescents and in adults there may be some fever and transient polyarthritis and polyarthralgia; very rarely encephalitis or thrombocytopenic purpura have been reported.

Outside epidemics, the disease is difficult to diagnose, for a similar type of rash may be caused by other viruses such as some of the enteroviruses.

## Epidemiology

The infection seems to spread from person to person mainly by the oropharyngeal route, but the period of infectivity appears to be short and rubella is not a highly infectious disease. It is not a notifiable disease and the two main sources of data on rubella infection in the UK are clinical reports by general practitioners to the Research Unit of the Royal College of Practitioners (Birmingham) and laboratory reports to the Communicable Disease Surveillance Centre (Colindale) which correlate fairly well.

Epidemics usually occur in the spring but, as may be seen from Figure 7, there is no clear periodicity. The disease does not appear to be as infectious as measles and, because predictable epidemics like those of measles (in the pre-vaccination days) do not occur, there has always been a varying proportion of susceptible adults in any population group.

## Congenital rubella

If a non-immune pregnant woman is infected with rubella virus the fetus may be at risk of infection, which may result in retardation of cell growth and necrosis. The earlier in pregnancy this occurs, the greater is the chance of severe congenital abnormalities, and the congenital rubella syndrome (CRS) may consist of single or multiple defects of the heart and great vessels, of the eyes and other organs. If all minor late defects and fetal deaths are included, the total risk of fetal damage after infection in the first 16 weeks of pregnancy is estimated at about 30–40%. The frequency is about 80% if infection occurs in the first 4 weeks of pregnancy, falling to 30–40%, 20% and 10% in the second, third and fourth months respectively. The true incidence is almost impossible to determine but useful information of any major changes should become apparent from the National Congenital Rubella Surveillance Programme (NCRSP) in the UK, which was set up in 1970, and the Collaborative Perinatal Research Study (CPRS) in the USA.

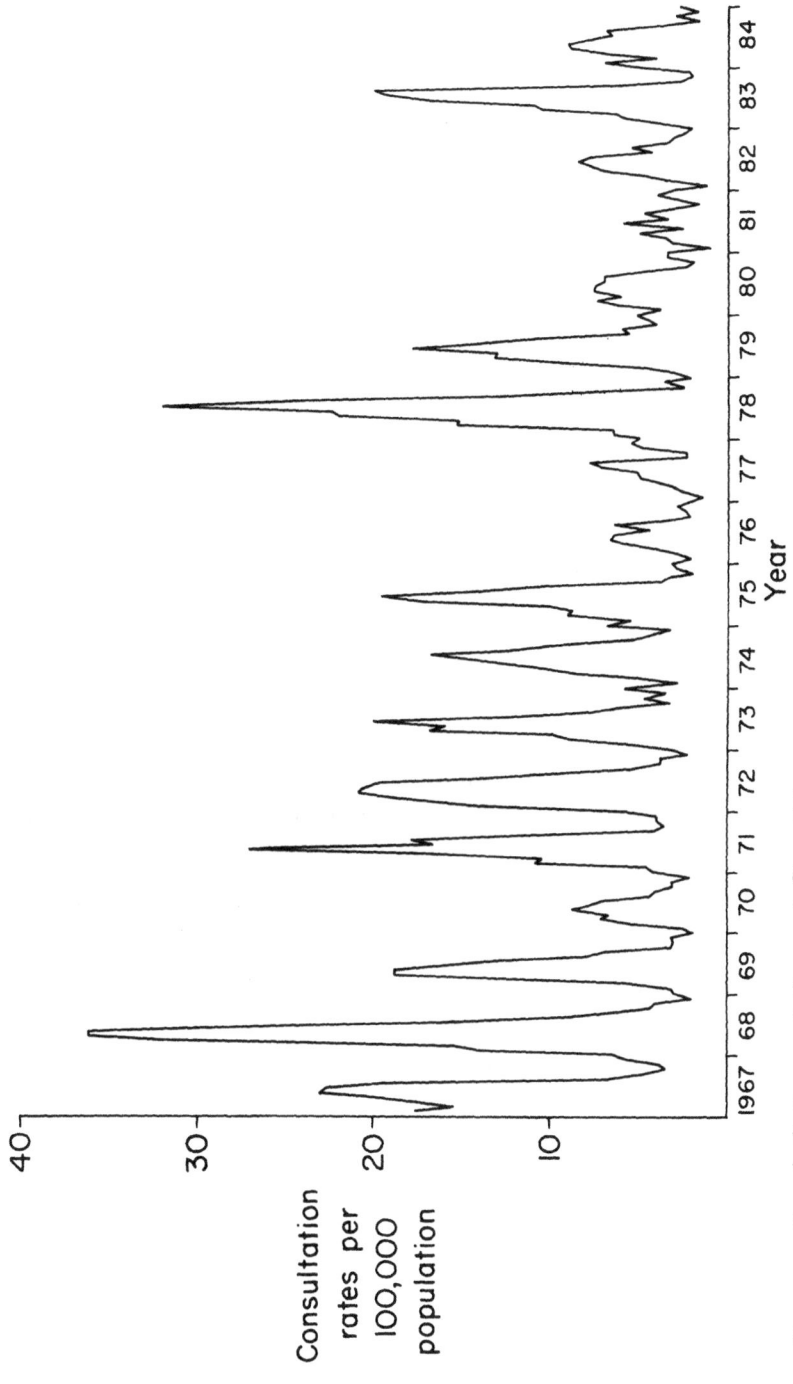

Source: Royal College of General Practitioners

**Figure 7** Rubella. Royal College of General Practitioners reports, United Kingdom 1967–84. (Prepared by CDSC)

In babies infected with no obvious damage, neurosensory deafness is common and occurs in about 15% of all cases of CRS.

In the UK, the confirmed or suspected cases of congenital rubella are shown in Table 15.

**Table 15**  Children with confirmed or suspected rubella by year of birth

| Year | Pre-1970 | 1970 | 71 | 72 | 73 | 74 | 75 | 76 | 77 | 78 | 79 | 1980 | 81 | 82 | 83 | All |
|------|----------|------|----|----|----|----|----|----|----|----|----|------|----|----|----|-----|
| Cases (*n*) | 96 | | 60 | 64 | 81 | 89 | 52 | 57 | 34 | 18 | 50 | 74 | 22 | 13 | 21 | 25 756 |

(From CDSC data)

In the USA prospective data from the CPRS indicate that, as a consequence of the 1964-5 epidemic, 30 000 children developed congenitally acquired rubella. In that epidemic, 3.6% of pregnant women had been infected compared with an infection rate of 0.1-0.2% in non-epidemic years.

There is a suggestion that the CRS may be proportionally more frequent in the infants of certain races, e.g. immigrants from the Indian subcontinent compared with UK residents. More information on the incidence of congenital rubella is required with regard to race and social class.

Of approximately 10 000 congenitally abnormal babies born each year in England and Wales only about 100-200 are caused by rubella.

Reinfections do not seem to be associated with detectable viraemia which would put a fetus at risk. If there is a rash and arthritis, viraemia should be assumed, with the possible attendant teratogenic effects.

## Rubella in women

It would appear from epidemiological and other data that about 80% of mothers are infected from their own children. There have, however, been considerable fluctuations over the years in the proportion of women infected in first pregnacies, but it appears that about 50% of congenitally abnormal live births are first born. The reason for this apparent discrepancy may be that many women infected during a first pregnancy had not gone to term.

The susceptibility of women appears to be variable and is dependent on race, social class and community. In the UK and USA before immunization was available about 15-20% of women of childbearing age appeared to be susceptible to rubella. However, antibody surveys in certain groups, e.g. student nurses, showed that as many as 40% may be susceptible.

In one study in young adults in the USA, 20% of those questioned did not know if they had had rubella: 80% knew they had, but half of them were wrong when their sera was tested. The rash is so fleeting that infection can take place unnoticed and, as already noted, a rubella-like rash may not be due to rubella virus. In the UK about 90% of women with no clinical history of rubella are immune and, in contrast, about 5% of women who think they have had rubella are devoid of antibodies. Because of the apparent relatively low infectivity of rubella it seems that only about one in ten susceptible women exposed to the disease becomes infected, either clinically or subclinically.

## Termination of pregnancies

In England and Wales between 1974 and 1981 for which data are available, there were 3273 terminations of pregnancies for rubella on *ground four* (i.e. a substantial risk of the baby being born abnormal) (Table 16). There is an additional category where termination may be indicated – namely, rubella immunization of a woman who was pregnant at the time of immunization or soon after. The number of these terminations between 1974 and 1977 was 27–40 a year, a figure to be compared with 156 in 1979, 101 in 1980 and 63 in 1981, which reflects the epidemic pattern of the disease (see Figure 7).

**Table 16** Termination for rubella (disease and contact), 1974–1981

| Year | All ages | < 20 y | % < 20 y |
|------|----------|--------|----------|
| 1974 | 633 | 54 | 8.5 |
| 1975 | 504 | 54 | 10.7 |
| 1976 | 213 | 18 | 8.4 |
| 1977 | 184 | 14 | 7.6 |
| 1978 | 830 | 53 | 6.4 |
| 1979 | 575 | 43 | 7.5 |
| 1980 | 200 | 24 | 12.0 |
| 1981 | 134 | 11 | 8.2 |
| All | 3273 | 271 | 8.3 |

It is estimated that of all terminations on *ground four*, about 60% are for maternal rubella, 20% in contacts and about 5-10% because they had inadvertently been given rubella vaccine.

There seems to have been a marked increase in recent years of the proportion of pregnacies terminated because of immunization during pregnancy, which may reflect the increased uptake of vaccine by women of childbearing age. A history of rubella infection may be inaccurate for, as noted, it is very difficult to diagnose clinically, especially if the disease occurs outside an epidemic period.

It is obvious that rubella causes a large fetal wastage and obviously much misery. At the same time it should be remembered that mere exposure to infection does not mean an abnormal fetus and only about one in ten of exposed susceptible women becomes infected.

Relatively simple laboratory tests are available which can provide evidence of a recent or past clinical or subclinical infection with rubella. The virus laboratory should be consulted in all cases where the termination of pregnancy is being considered.

## Vaccines

At the present time, only live virus vaccines are available, which are prepared from the RA 27/3 or from the Cendehill attenuated strains of rubella virus. The former was isolated from a rubella-infected conceptus and grown in WI-38 human diploid cells and the latter virus from the urine of a patient with acute rubella and grown in rabbit-kidney tissue cultures. Although both these viruses have been recovered from the nasopharynx of immunized individuals, studies of more than 1200 household contacts have yielded no convincing evidence of person-to-person spread of vaccine virus and the possibility of transmission of virus to susceptible close contacts is such a remote possibility that it can be regarded as irrelevant.

The RA 27/3 vaccine appears to be more likely than other vaccines to induce an immune response which is qualitatively comparable to that following the natural disease and is in this respect preferable. Some studies have suggested that the Cendehill strain produces fewer reactions in young women, but as these are generally mild this is not important. Antibody titres after vaccination are usually about four to eight times lower than those following a natural infection.

The vaccine is issued as freeze-dried preparation to be reconstituted before use with distilled water which is supplied with the vaccine. It should be given by deep subcutaneous injection as soon as possible after reconstitution. Vaccine and diluent should be stored in the cool part of the refrigerator (about $+4\,°C$) but should not be frozen as the ampoule may crack.

## Vaccine strategies

When rubella vaccine became available for routine use in 1969, the objective was clear – namely, to prevent the congenital rubella syndrome (CRS). A direct approach to this was not possible for (1) there was little evidence of the possible adverse effect of vaccine virus on the fetus, (2) the possibility of person-to-person spread of vaccine had not been eliminated with the potential danger of pregnant house-hold contacts of vaccinated children being at risk and (3) the durability of vaccine-induced immunity and the possibility of preventing transmission by mass vaccination of children was uncertain.

In the UK a programme of selective immunization of girls of 12–14 years of age (subsequently 10–14) was proposed with the intention of ensuring protection of the fetus (if and when they became pregnant). It was hoped that with this scheme, the 'wild' virus would continue to circulate in the community and boost the vaccine-induced immunity. It was realized that with such a scheme several years would elapse before there was any evidence that it would reduce the incidence of the CRS. Accordingly, it was decided to extend this scheme to immunize girls of 16–19 years of age and indeed to ensure that all seronegative women were immunized, with particular reference to 'screening' of all pregnant women for evidence of antibody during their antenatal care and immunization of those devoid of antibody *after* delivery.

In the USA an effort has been made to immunize *all* children, with the assumption that vaccine-induced immunity is durable and that transmission of rubella virus will be interrupted and the disease eradicated.

The various assumptions which determined these strategies have now been resolved: (1) although vaccine virus can infect the fetus there is no evidence that it has *ever* caused congenital rubella, (2) there is no evidence of transmission of vaccine virus to contacts and (3) the vaccine appears to have a more than 90% efficacy and to provide protection for at least 10 years and possibly for life.

So far, the results of the UK policy to prevent the CRS have been disappointing, although the full effect of the schoolgirl and subsidiary programmes have not had enough time to be assessed. The uptake of vaccine by schoolgirls has with some exceptions been poor. In Edinburgh (Lothian Health District) it has been possible for Dr Zealley and her colleagues to achieve a 97% acceptance rate. The method should be followed in other areas. Girls are tested for antibody by radial haemolysis from capillary blood and those who are susceptible (27%) are then immunized and again tested for antibody by a capillary blood test. This very high rate of acceptance in school-girls requires co-operation of the Community Child Health Service with the laboratory, with schools and a dedicated team of health care personnel. It also has a spin-off in vaccine acceptance in older women, which has been generally poor in women of childbearing age. There is no doubt that in some areas the school and adult vaccination programmes have reduced the number of women in the childbearing age who are susceptible to rubella, but during outbreaks the risk of infection of susceptible women during pregnancy is still high.

In the UK the strategy was good, the tactics have with a few exceptions been poor. The reasons for this, some of which apply to the acceptance of other routine immunizations (see Figure 8) are multiple:

(1) the divided responsibility for ensuring that immunization is done – who takes responsibility and action on receipt of a CMO (DHSS Chief Medical Officer) letter on immunization addressed to General Medical Practitioners, District Medical Officer, District Nursing Officers with copies to Regional Medical Officers etc?

(2) the lack of communication between laboratories which do screening, hospitals, clinics, general practitioners, obstetricians and other hospital doctors,

(3) confusion between screening and immunization,

(4) the absence or lack of availability of adequate records,

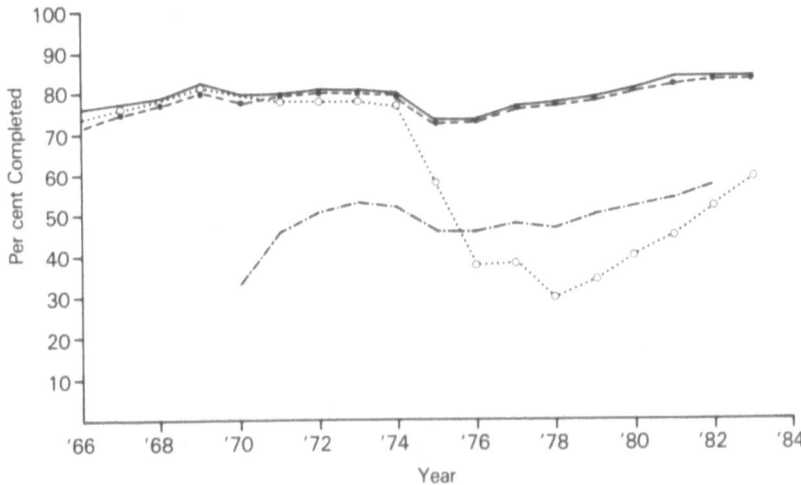

**Figure 8** Immunization - England and Wales. Acceptance rates, percentage of children completed immunization by end of second year after birth (from DHSS data). ———— = dip and tetanus (tet from 1968); --●-- = polio; ···○··· = pertussis; −·−·− = measles (1970: 9 months only)

(5) the generally poor standard of health education and the in-efficacy of central government exhortation,

(6) with the exception of a few general practitioners the apparent lack of *any* mission of all those involved, to ensure that they 'have got their act together'.

Personally, I cannot see any hope for much improvement in the acceptance of rubella and other vaccines in the UK unless some action is taken with respect to items 1–6 listed above.

In the United States, tactics of administering 123 million doses of vaccine since 1969 have prevented epidemics of rubella and CRS from occurring. Recently there has been a further decline in the incidence of rubella in adolescents and in the number of cases of congenital rubella. This is in part due to increased coverage of older children at high schools and doubtless, as with measles immunization in the USA, immunization against rubella will become a requirement for school and college entry.

Everyone involved in the rubella immunization programme has to ask if we are achieving the objective of preventing the CRS. It must be appreciated that at the present time, while pregnancy is a theoretical risk to rubella immunization, if vaccination occurs in pregnancy 'the risk of vaccine associated malformations is so small as to be negligible' and it 'should not be a reason to *routinely* recommend interruption of pregnancy'. At the same time, until more data are collected pregnant women should not be vaccinated.

What about screening? Many women do not understand that, when blood is taken for 'screening', this is a test for immunity; many of them think that they have been immunized, but, furthermore, the transmission of the result of the test and the recall system do not always operate effectively. I have not seen an accurate study on the cost-effectiveness of rubella immunization with and without 'screening', but it *should be* cost-effective to screen capillary blood and test it by radio-immune haemolysis.

It is important to be able to tell a woman who has been vaccinated and who has soon after become pregnant that she was naturally immune before immunization and need not be concerned about the *theoretical risk* of vaccine damage to her fetus.

I would like to see general practitioners assume greater responsibility for ensuring that all women in their practices are protected against rubella. Some have achieved this – but there are problems of mobility of patients, particularly in the inner conurbations. To ensure adequate coverage I believe that there must be the fullest co-operation between the general practitioner and the school health service which should ensure that *all* girls are screened for antibody at 10 years of age and immunized if necessary, and immunized again at 15 years of age or at school leaving if not tested for antibody after the first immunization. (This would ensure that a vaccine with a 90% effectiveness would give a greater than 90% protection and reduce vaccine failures.)

Secondly, I believe, general practitioners should ensure that *all* non-pregnant women of childbearing age in their practices were screened and immunized and given advice on contraception for 3 months after immunization. Thirdly, Health Visitors should become responsible for ensuring that all susceptible pregnant women are immunized postpartum. This programme could be modified with further evidence of the absence of risk to the fetus of the presently available vaccines. Immunization of a person who is already immune as a result of a previous infection or immunization presents no hazard. A call for 90% immunization is not acceptable – the objective must be 100%.

Priority in immunization of adults should be given to nurses and nursery staff, particularly those in health centres, general practices, paediatric, antenatal and obstetric units and medical students, not only for protection of these categories but to minimize the chance of their transmitting rubella to pregnant women. Male doctors working in units dealing with pregnant women should also be immunized, as also should women teachers in schools and in teacher training colleges.

## Reactions

The administration of vaccine may be followed by mild symptoms such as fever, rash, lymphadenopathy or occasionally a sore throat, but such complications appear to be rare. The only really troublesome adverse reactions reported have been arthralgia, which occurs in approximately 25% of vaccinated females, and arthritis with pain and stiffness in the fingers, cervical spine, knees and ankles, which occurs in about 1% of them. Both these reactions increase with age and are uncommon in children. It seems sensible to advise very active females, such as physical education instructors and physiotherapists, to take things easy for about a fortnight after immunization. Any adverse reactions to the vaccine should be reported.

## Contraindications

An absolute contraindication is pregnancy. There is no contraindication of vaccinating a seropositive woman. Other contraindications are similar to those outlined under measles vaccine.

## Inactivated virus

Little progress with an inactivated rubella virus vaccine has as yet been reported. The development of such a vaccine is called for and it would solve many of the problems of preventing the CRS. It could be given as a combined polyvalent vaccine with boosters if required.

## Combined vaccines

Combinations of live measles/mumps/rubella (MMR), measles/rubella and rubella/mumps vaccines have been recently licensed in the

USA and appear to be effective. The MMR vaccine has been introduced routinely in some places at 1 year of age. It appears to give very
good serological conversion rates and should provide a hope of greatly
limiting the transmission of each of the diseases in communities with
high vaccine coverage. The advantage of MMR is that it simplifies the
introduction of mumps vaccine without interfering with the acceptance of measles and rubella vaccines and could provide better overall
protection against the three diseases.

# 9
# Tuberculosis

Although tuberculosis has shown a continuing decline since the earliest statistics were available, it still causes more deaths than any other notifiable disease. It is caused by *Mycobacterium tuberculosis* (the tubercle bacillus) but immunization with the attenuated tubercle bacillus BCG (Bacille Calmette-Guérin), plays only a minor part in the control of the disease in most situations.

## *Mycobacterium tuberculosis*

There are three types of mycobacteria which cause the disease: (1) *M. tuberculosis*, (2) *M. bovis* and (3) a number of atypical mycobacteria. They are rod shaped bacteria which do not stain well but when they do, they resist decolorization and are therefore called 'acid fast' bacilli. They grow on a variety of culture media but at a much slower rate than most other bacteria and they are generally more resistant to chemical agents.

## Tuberculosis

*M. tuberculosis* may infect many organs but the commonest disease is pulmonary tuberculosis, and there may be dissemination of bacteria to lymph nodes and spread throughout the body. *M. bovis* usually causes an alimentary infection which may also become widespread.

The tubercle bacillus is highly infectious for most individuals. A very few who are exposed to infection show no indication of having acquired the disease and they remain susceptible; about 95–98% of those infected do not develop any clinically significant disease. As is well known, after infection a small focus forms at the site of primary lodgement of the bacilli in the lungs or in the alimentary tract. The organisms multiply and produce a granuloma which results in the development of cell mediated immunity and the individual becomes sensitized to tuberculin protein and 'immune'. For the great majority this is the end of the story, for a few there is limited local spread in lymph glands, lungs, brain, bone and joints. In most instances the defence mechanism of the body can respond and control these foci but they may extend and cause extensive destruction of tissues. Much of the clinical disease involving the chest or abdomen occurs within a year after infection, as does tuberculous meningitis and miliary tuberculosis. Although the spread of infection becomes limited, some bacteria will remain encased in the primary focus and may be awakened after many years by a decline in the defence mechanism of the host. In some cases, the disease in adults is due to reinfection.

## Epidemiology

Apart from transmission by milk from infected cows, which is now largely controlled in most countries by pasteurization and slaughter of infected animals, human tuberculosis is spread from person to person by droplet infection. There are many factors which determine the prevalence of the disease, such as family size, overcrowding, malnutrition etc, which facilitate the aerosol spread of the bacteria. As with many other infective diseases, tuberculosis reached its peak during the industrial revolution with the growth of towns and migration into them from the country districts. During that period, the

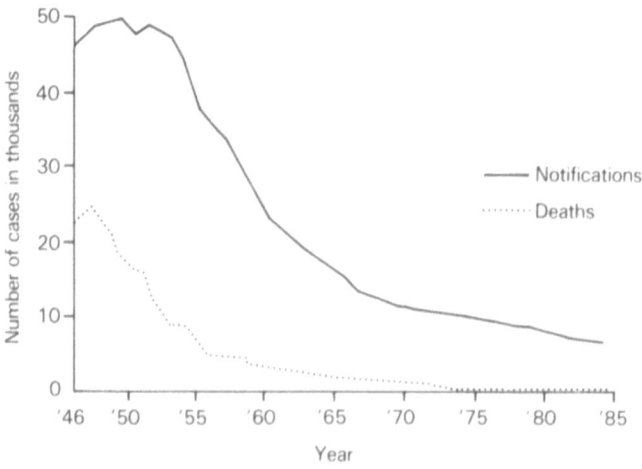

**Figure 9**  Tuberculosis notifications and deaths, England and Wales

annual mortality rates from tuberculosis were probably in the region of 1%. The introduction of BCG (1925) had little influence on mortality, but a dramatic decline occurred with the introduction of chemotherapy in the 1940s.

The annual rate of decline in mortality over the years (Figure 9) has been markedly different in the various age groups and in males as compared with females (Figures 10 and 11). At present, deaths from tuberculosis in the UK occur essentially in males over 45 years of age, and in recent years over 90% of deaths from all forms of tuberculosis (mainly respiratory tuberculosis) have been in that age group. About 20% of all these deaths occurred in patients in whom tuberculosis was diagnosed only *after* death and many might have been prevented by better use of the facilities available for diagnosis and treatment.

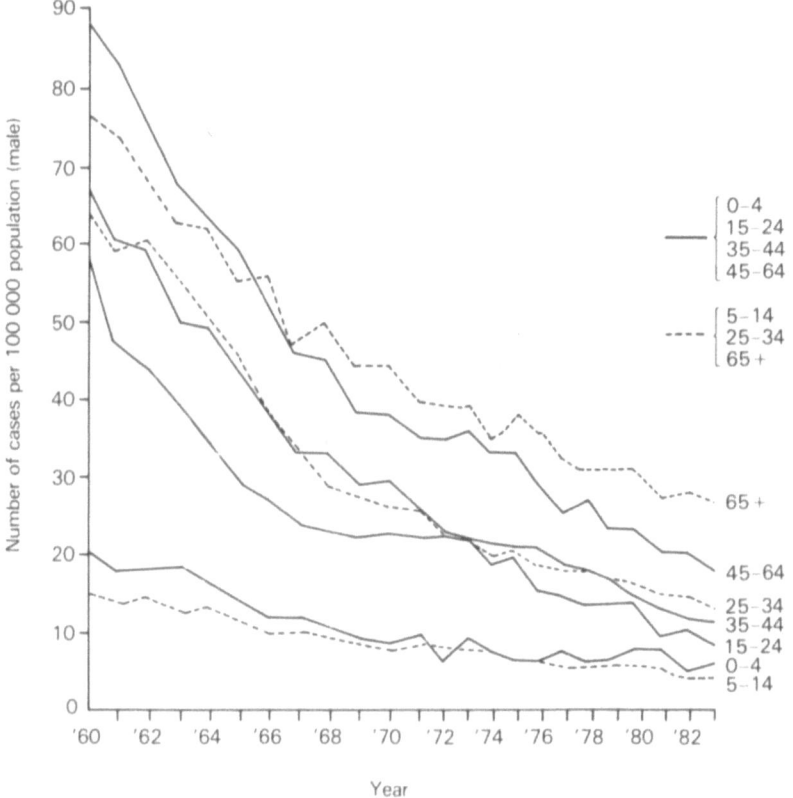

**Figure 10**  Tuberculosis of the respiratory system. Notification rates per 100 000 population (males), England and Wales

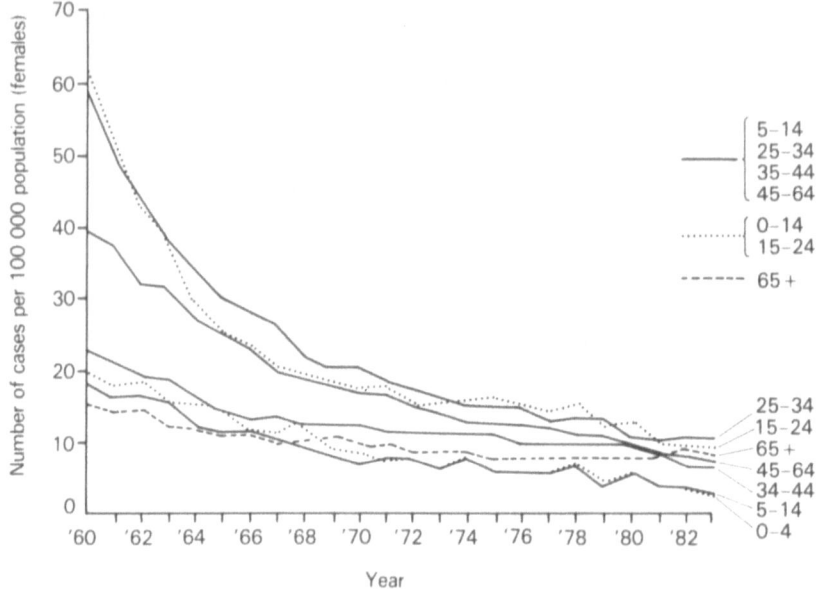

**Figure 11** Tuberculosis of the respiratory system. Notifcation rates per 100 000 population (females), England and Wales

## Notifications

Notifications (Figure 10) did not start to decline significantly until 1954, and even with improved ascertainment there was little decline in prevalence comparable to that of mortality.

Notifications, although not an accurate index of the incidence of the disease, are a more reliable index of the present epidemiological situation of tuberculosis than mortality statistics. However, notifications do not give a clear picture of the incidence of the disease because they indicate neither the onset nor the time of infection. The importance of notifying tuberculosis is that it helps to ensure immediate investigation of possible sources of infection.

In 1972 the national rates for all forms of tuberculosis in England and Wales were 22.8 per 100 000 population. These rates vary from area to area, reflecting urbanization and the socioeconomic conditions of several decades as well as of today. The reduction of tuberculosis has slowed down in some areas, apparently because of immigration. A recent survey in England demonstrated that 32% of notified cases were in persons born outside the UK. The rate is said to be 27 and 54 times higher respectively for those born in India and Pakistan than for those born in England and Wales. Between 1965 and 1971 there was a decrease in notifications of about 7% per year among those born in Africa, India and Pakistan.

## History

Although Koch's discovery of *M. tuberculosis* in 1882 did not have any obvious effect on the control of the disease, it led to an understanding of the hypersensitivity response when live or dead *M. tuberculosis* was injected into tuberculous animals and to the development of the tuberculin test which is not only used as a diagnostic test in individuals exposed to tuberculosis (for surveillance and for epidemiological surveys), but also for the selection of individuals for immunization with BCG.

## Tuberculin test

The test requires careful standardization and dosage because most people will respond if a sufficiently large amount of tuberculin is injected. Of the various types of tuberculin tests the intradermal (Mantoux) or multiple puncture (Heaf) are the most accurate and the most commonly used and may be carried out with old tuberculin, but purified protein derivatives of tuberculin (PPD) are now commonly used.

## Mantoux test

In the Mantoux test a convenient dose is 10 tuberculin units (TU) in 0.1 ml of buffer solution or saline injected intradermally with a very short (6 mm, 26 gauge) needle, usually into the left forearm using a special disposable tuberculin syringe marked in 0.1 ml divisions (1 TU = 0.002 mg of dried PPD).

## Reactions

If the injection has been given properly a wheal of about 8 mm is raised which disappears within a couple of hours. Sometimes there is an immediate reaction of oedema and erythema which appears within

15 minutes of injection. This is followed by the characteristic delayed reaction which appears in most individuals with previous experience with mycobacteria. The time of its appearance and its extent give a measure of the degree of sensitivity of the individual. The reaction is usually at its maximum between 48 and 72 hours after the injection and consists of a central area of induration and erythema of variable diameter. In making a quantitative assessment of the test reaction, only the area of induration which can be felt and seen is measured. The reaction is usually graded as negative when there is no induration even if erythema is present. Only reactions with a diameter of 6 mm or more are acceptable as evidence of previous mycobacterial infection. A strongly positive reaction may be defined as 15 mm or more induration and should be referred for further investigation and supervision. A reaction of 20 mm or more is regarded as severe. Since it may be indicative of a tuberculous lesion somewhere in the body, individuals developing severe reactions should be given a thorough clinical and X-ray examination. If clear, it should be repeated after 6 months. (It must be remembered that tuberculosis can infect areas other than the lungs.) A general reaction with fever accompanying a Mantoux reaction of 15 mm or more is a strong indication of an active lesion somewhere in the body. If there is no reaction, this indicates that the person has no tuberculous lesion in his body. Individuals with immunological deficiencies or those suffering from serious illnesses may also have a non-reactor state (i.e. tuberculin anergy) which is also present in the newborn and in the aged. The tuberculin reaction also becomes negative after an attack of measles or after measles immunization, and also in infectious mononucleosis. It is depressed in active leprosy and in sarcoidosis and in patients receiving steroid therapy.

## Heaf test

The Heaf test employs a simple and rapid technique in which a punch (the Heaf 'gun'), which has a ring of six solid needles, is released to a depth of 1 mm through a drop of full strength PPD or tuberculin containing 100 000 units per ml. (This must not be used for Mantoux tests unless diluted to 10 units/ml.) The drop should be placed on the arm with a sterilized glass rod or dropper and spread over with the end plate of the gun.

## Reactions

The reactions to the Heaf test are read in 4–10 days (although positive results may appear earlier). If the result is negative there is no erythema or puncture marks nor any induration. In a normal healthy individual this response indicates that consideration may be given to immunize with BCG. In a grade I response there are easily palpable discrete papules round some of the puncture points and this type of response is usually classified as 'tuberculin negative' and the individual may be immunized unless this has been previously done. (Some consider that a grade I response which fades by 3 or 4 days is non-specific and that a grade I response at 7 days is indicative of infection.) With grade II there is a coalescence of indurated papules to form a ring and in grade III a wheal with induration, while in grade IV there is a greater reaction than in grade III, with a blister or central haemorrhage. Grades II, III and IV responders should be referred for clinical examination and X-ray, except in the case of grade II responders who have previously been immunized with BCG.

## Tuberculin sensitivity

It is now realized that low grade tuberculin sensitivity is partly tuberculous in origin and partly the result of natural infections with non-tuberculous strains of mycobacteria (including avian strains) and various atypical bacteria. Similarly, subclinical infections with atypical mycobacteria may result in enhanced resistance to subsequent infection with *M. tuberculosis* and individuals who show a low grade reactivity to tuberculin (reacting to only 100 TU) have a lower incidence of tuberculosis in follow-up than do tuberculin negative individuals. While there is a relationship between the degree of the reaction and the strength of the dose of tuberculin, of more practical importance is the fact that the degree of sensitivity gives some indication of the activity of an infection and the risk of subsequent complications and relapse. In England, children with a strongly positive result, i.e. an induration of 15 mm or more to 3 TU, were shown in a Medical Research Council trial to have had an annual rate of tuberculosis of 2.93 per 1000 during the first 2½ years of the trial compared with 0.78 among those with 5–14 mm induration.

The tuberculin test provides an accurate index of the incidence of the disease and, e.g., study of the numbers of tuberculin positive children from year to year in different ages and classes in schools has also given a valuable index of a source of infection to which a particular class has been exposed.

## Control

Preventive measures depend on:

(1)　detection of cases and their treatment,

(2)　the examination of contacts including tuberculin testing and chest radiology,

(3)　BCG vaccination,

(4)　health education.

It would seem sensible to tuberculin test (and X-ray) all immigrants (see page 96) from countries with a high incidence of tuberculosis. Such a procedure could be compulsory on their arrival to initiate treatment and prevent spread in the community. Although the disease may not become clinically manifest in immigrants until a few years after arrival, identification on arrival could initiate immediate treatment and surveillance of contacts.

## Immunization

Soon after tuberculin had been discovered and it had been demonstrated that tuberculous individuals showed increased sensitivity (Koch phenomenon), Robert Koch (1890) claimed that 'tuberculin' could be used for treatment of early cases. However, this was soon discredited, as was vaccination with other inactive preparations. It became clear that dead bacilli or extracts of mycobacteria would not stimulate immunity and that in order to be protected against tuberculosis it was necessary to have experienced an infection. This may be achieved by BCG which undergoes a limited growth in human tissues and produces sensitivity and increased resistance to subsequent infection.

# BCG

BCG was derived from a bovine strain of *M. tuberculosis* by Calmette and Guérin (1906). They observed that when bile was added to the medium in which the bacteria were grown, clumps of the micro-organisms became dispersed and changes occurred in their morphology and virulence. They postulated that prolonged subculture in such a bile-containing medium might produce an attenuated vaccine strain. After 231 subcultures over a period of 13 years the resulting strain was found to be harmless to man.

When BCG vaccine was introduced in the 1920s it was widely used in France where it was given orally. Although vaccination was popular, there were no statistically controlled trials and many considered the procedure unsafe. In 1930 BCG received a setback (as does practically every new vaccine) with the Lübeck disaster in which 73 infants (27%) who had been fed the vaccine died. It was apparent that the children had accidentally been fed with a virulent strain of *M. tuberculosis* which had been kept in the same laboratory as the stock of BCG strain. The disaster led to regulations controlling the production of BCG to ensure exclusion of all other strains. The WHO Expert Committee on Tuberculosis has repeatedly warned against the multiplication of laboratories preparing BCG vaccine; in the UK the vaccine is produced by only one commercial firm and the entire production process is rigorously monitored.

## *Administration*

Inactivation of liquid BCG vaccine occurs readily on exposure to light and to tropical temperatures and the development of freeze-dried vaccine, now in common use, which maintains its potency for at least 12 months if kept at $+4\,^{\circ}C$ has increased the efficacy of BCG in tropical countries.

The vaccine is usually given by intradermal (i.d.) injection. The freeze-dried vaccine is reconstituted in saline (which is supplied with the vaccine) and it should be used immediately after reconstitution and kept out of sunlight. The skin at the site of vaccination should be cleaned with ether or acetone but not with an antiseptic. 0.1 ml of the vaccine is injected into the skin just above the insertion of the deltoid with a 1 ml disposable syringe with a short-bevel 25 gauge needle, raising a wheal of about 8 mm. If BCG is administered too high, or too far forward or backward, the adjacent lymph glands (infraclavicular, cephalic, cervical or axillary) may become involved and tender. (Complications seem to be more common if the injection is given into the skin of the thigh.)

After about 1 week a red papule appears at the injection site and this increases in size for 2–3 weeks to about 1 cm in diameter or to a benign ulcer which heals in 6–12 weeks leaving a small scar. No dressing should be used unless there is much discharge from the ulcer, in which case a dry dressing should suffice.

The vaccine may also be given by multiple puncture using a Heaf gun; in this case papules which are variable in number appear at the sites of punctures about a week after vaccination. They seldom show any obvious ulceration and heal with nearly invisible scars in about 10 weeks. This technique gives consistently good conversion which, although slightly less than that obtained by i.d. injections, is suitable for use by less skilled people.

There is no point in doing a tuberculin test in infants prior to BCG vaccination because this test is never positive in the first few weeks of life, even in babies of tuberculous mothers. With babies, great care must be taken to ensure that the inoculation is given intradermally and not subcutaneously which may give rise to a persistent local reaction. The dosage for infants is 0.05 ml.

## Abnormal reactions

Faulty injection technique is the most frequent cause of severe reactions which may be local, regional or general. There may be excessive ulceration at the site of inoculation. This is best treated with a dry gauze dressing, daily, until the granulating surface is clean, then with application twice weekly of 3% tetracycline ointment. Shallow ulcers with markedly undercut edges are slow to heal and healing is helped by application every other day of a solution of dimethyl sulphoxide to the raw surface and especially under the loose overhanging skin edge, followed by a compression dressing of gauze and bandage. This helps the loose skin to survive and stick to the underlying raw area. Once this has happened, application of 3% tetracycline ointment will prevent gauze sticking to the remaining ulcer and healing will quickly follow.

'BCG lupus', eczema and hypertropic scars and keloid formation have been described following vaccination with BCG. The former is a persistent granuloma which always heals but often very slowly. Keloid is unusual in Europe but is said to occur with 'alarming' frequency in Israel.

An abscess may develop at the inoculation site. This is usually due to too large a dose or too deep an injection. These abscesses are usually sterile and heal rapidly once the necrotic material has been drained.

Lymphangitis and severe adenitis (with or without caseation) may follow a misplaced injection, but mild regional adenitis is so common following vaccination that it can be regarded as normal. In severe reactions showing streaks of lymphangitis there is sometimes a tendency to administer antibiotics or antihistamine. These are said not to help, but the application of 2% steroid ointment may be of value. Adenitis is less frequent after vaccination by multiple puncture with the Heaf gun.

General untoward reactions are rare. About 15 fatalities following BCG, due to widespread dissemination of the organism, have been reported in the world literature; most if not all of them have occurred in individuals with immunological abnormalities.

## Successful vaccination

Successful vaccination may be judged by conversion to a moderate positive Mantoux reaction, 3-4 weeks after vaccination. This conversion is often slower in young babies, but it should occur in 100% of those vaccinated with potent vaccine.

## Evaluation of vaccines

Although the UK was about the last country to introduce immunization as a routine measure, the best trial of BCG which is being carried out in England, involving more than 50 000 schoolchildren and which was started in 1950, shows that after 15 years the protective efficacy appears to be about 70%. This was similar in both sexes and extended to all forms of tuberculosis. It rose to a peak at 2½-5 years after vaccination and then decreased.

In other parts of the world the efficacy of BCG has varied (Table 17) from nil in a trial in Georgia schoolchildren (1947), and 31% in Puerto Rican schoolchildren (1940-51) to approximately 80% protection in American Indians (1935-8). Recently (1968), in the largest controlled field trial which has ever been done (carried out in Southern India), the vaccine appeared to have no protective effect.

**Table 17**  Rate of tuberculosis and protection afforded by BCG in various populations

| | Tuberculosis in unvaccinated (per 1000 per year) | Protection from BCG (percentages) |
|---|---|---|
| N. American Indians | 15.6 | 80 |
| Chicago infants | 2.2 | 75 |
| British schoolchildren | 1.3 | 78 |
| S. Indian rural population | 0.86 | 60 |
| Puerto Rican children | 0.43 | 31 |
| Georgian (Alabama) population | 0.13 | 14 |
| Georgian schoolchildren | 0.11 | 0 |

(From Sutherland, J. (1971) Tubercle, **53**, 10)

There has been much controversy as to the efficacy of BCG and very discrepant results have been reported from different countries. Although some trial results have seriously questioned its efficacy, BCG has continued to be used extensively in many countries.

The existence of non-tuberculous mycobacterial infections in man and their immunological interaction with *M. tuberculosis* and BCG at the level of protective immunity and delayed-type hypersensitivity has helped to explain the apparent discrepancies in the tests of the effectiveness of BCG.

At the same time differences in the vaccine (e.g. lyophilized or fluid), differences in the local strains of *M. tuberculosis*, the prevalence of infected individuals and the socioeconomic conditions of the community where the trials have been done may be some of the factors underlying the differences which have been observed in the efficacy of BCG in various parts of the world. Trials showing lack of efficacy in one situation must not lead to the conclusion that BCG offers no protection against tuberculosis in any situation.

# Who should be immunized?

The great disadvantage of BCG is the loss of the tuberculin test as an indicator of a natural infection by tuberile bacilli.

## *Routine immunization in the UK*

At the present time BCG is recommended for schoolchildren between their 10th and 14th birthday, if found to be tuberculin negative. I have long believed that it should be abandoned as a routine procedure throughout the UK as it has now been in some districts.

It has been estimated that in England between 1970 and 1980 the annual incidence of tuberculosis in unvaccinated subjects will be between 0.04 and 0.1 per 1000. These estimates are just below the lowest figure (0.11) in Table 17. It might be expected that in the future, routine BCG vaccination in the UK will make virtually no contribution to the reduction of tuberculosis.

Furthermore, it has been calculated that in the UK, the routine use of BCG in 13-year-olds in the 1970s would reduce the annual notification rate for negatives from about one to less than 0.2 per 10 000, i.e. vaccinating 10 000 children might prevent ten cases in the next 10 years. By the 1980s, the reduction in notifications through using BCG was estimated at about 0.4 per 10 000 per year. This means that about four cases could be prevented in the following 10 years by vaccination of 10 000 13-year-olds. By the late 1980s the vaccination of 10 000 13-year-olds will prevent only one case in the following 10 years. Obviously, *routine* BCG immunization in the UK is not based on risk–cost-effectiveness ratios and, as in the case of smallpox vaccine, it will be abandoned for political reasons long after it is obvious that medically it should no longer be recommended as a routine procedure.

## *Selective immunization in the UK*

BCG should be offered to those living in crowded conditions in urban communities, and to all immigrants and their children from countries with a high incidence of tuberculosis.

All hospital workers who come into contact with patients, i.e. doctors, nurses, medical students, laboratory staff and necropsy attendants should be given a tuberculin test. In Europe it is usually recommended that all those who are tuberculin negative or weakly positive should be given BCG. In the USA there is a strong body of opinion that such individuals should be kept under regular medical supervision and be periodically tuberculin tested; I subscribe to that view.

All persons going to work in developing countries of high prevalence of the disease should be offered vaccine if tuberculin negative.

All contacts of known cases of tuberculosis should be vaccinated. With children it is customary to tuberculin-test the child, and if negative to remove the child from contact where possible and then vaccinate following a second tuberculin test. The reason for the second test is to minimize the possibility that the child is naturally infected at the time of the tuberculin test. If the child was infected prior to the first test, the result might be negative because allergy had not developed. Babies should be similarly treated but without prior tuberculin testing. Tuberculin conversion may be detected by 6 weeks after vaccination; ideally, possible contacts should therefore be segregated from exposure for that time. If segregation is not possible, and if isoniazid is to be given prophylactically, the use of isoniazid-resistant BCG should be considered for their immunization.

High risk group individuals who have been vaccinated in the past but have reverted to being tuberculin negative may be revaccinated.

## Contraindications

Positive reactors should not be vaccinated nor should children with a known immunological abnormality. Those suffering from any infectious disease, e.g. measles or whooping cough, or receiving corticosteroids or other immunosuppressive drugs should not be given BCG. As noted, weak positive reactions are no longer regarded as a contraindication to vaccination.

Although there is no evidence of ill effects from BCG vaccination in pregnant mothers, it should be avoided except in situations of very high risk of infection of the mother during the pregnancy.

BCG has been given at the same time as other live and inactive vaccines but in general it seems wiser to allow an interval of 3 weeks between the administration of two live vaccines.

## General measures

Although in decline, tuberculosis is still an important and common disease in the industrialized countries, where detection of cases and examination of contacts and chemoprophylaxis are more important for the future control of this disease than vaccination.

# 10
# Vaccines for Selective Use

## INFLUENZA

Influenza epidemics are caused by a virus of which there are three types, A, B and C. Although a great deal is known about the viruses, prevention of the disease by immunization has up to the present, been of limited success.

## The disease

One certain fact about influenza is that it is an epidemic virus disease involving the upper respiratory system. There are all grades of severity, but 'influenza' is probably the most abused clinical diagnosis and is applied to all sorts of upper respiratory infections, pyrexias of unknown origin and various alimentary upsets. (Outbreaks of 'gastric flu', in summer or autumn, whatever they may be caused by, are not due to influenza virus as recognized.) This does not mean that an outbreak of influenza cannot occur in the autumn and it may be the harbinger of a more widespread winter epidemic. Influenza has a widespread spectrum of signs and symptoms, but classically it is characterized by an abrupt onset of fever, headache, aches in the limbs, and respiratory tract catarrh often with a hoarse cough.

Influenza is highly contagious and one should be very sceptical in diagnosing influenza in isolated cases or individual family outbreaks.

## The viruses

Influenza A, B and C viruses belong to the family of orthomyxoviridae. Some clues to the natural history of influenza epidemics have come from studies of the structure of these viruses which have a ribonucleic acid core which consists not of one single molecule, as in related myxo-viruses, but of five discrete segments, and the great mutability of influenza viruses is presumably related to this. Surrounding the nucleoprotein is the viral envelope on the surface of which are two types of glycoprotein spikes, one of which is a haemagglutinin (H) and the other which functions as a neuraminidase enzyme (N).

The haemagglutinin haemagglutinates the red cells of some species *in vitro* because there happen to be specific complementary receptor sites on the red cells and on the virus particles. The ability to haemagglutinate forms the basis of an important test for studying the presence of antibody and for testing sera to determine the relationship of one influenza virus to another. If the antibody is specific to the particular virus, it will 'neutralize' the virus receptor and haemagglutination will not occur – so-called 'haemagglutination inhibition'. The haemagglutinin appears to be the most important antigen in stimulating protective immunity. The neuraminidase may act on mucoproteins of the respiratory secretions and facilitate contact of virus and cell. More importantly, it may determine the amount of virus released by a given cell.

The viruses are grouped into types A, B, C on the basis of the distinct antigenic characters of the internal components. Because of the split genome, genetic reassortment can readily take place not only with viruses of their own type (with a possibility of $2^8$ ( $= 256$) different combinations) but, as influenza A virus infects pigs, horses, birds and fish as well as man, reassortment (sometimes referred to as recombination) can also occur with animal viruses in nature. Viruses of influenza type A are further divided into subtypes on the basis of the haemagglutinin and neuraminidase antigens which gives rise to the nomenclature of influenza A viruses, such as H1N1 or H3N2.

## Epidemiology

Influenza A virus is responsible for widespread epidemics which occur every few years and major worldwide pandemics about every 10–20 years. It seems that these major pandemics are caused by viruses to which the host population has not been previously exposed. The pandemics wane as more of the susceptible persons in the population become immune and the pandemic strain is then replaced by a 'new' virus showing an 'antigenic *shift*' and very different from the previous pandemic virus, and another pandemic occurs. These 'new' viruses seem to arise by gradual changes ('antigenic *drifts*') which give rise to epidemics which occur between the pandemic years.

'Antigenic *shift*' seems to occur so suddenly and the 'new virus' spreads so rapidly that it seems to be unlikely to be entirely due to mutation and selection which can explain 'antigenic *drift*' a process which can be reproduced in the laboratory. This is not possible with 'antigenic shifts'. Many theories have been proposed to explain the origin of 'new' influenza A viruses, from transfer of viruses from animals to man, from parasites to man, or from man to man following reactivation of a virus which had circulated many years previously in an infective form and then gone 'latent' and non-productive for many years. It has also been proposed that virus reservoirs in man or animals might be activated by solar radiation and also that 'new' viruses could come from outer space!

In 1427 in the reign of Henry VI, an unknown chronicler in St Albans wrote, 'Quaedam infirmatas reumigata invasit totum populum . . . et sic senes cum junioribus inficiebat quod magnum numerum ad funus letale deducebat'. This states the essential features of an influenza epidemic and implies the sudden outbreak of a widespread infection with the highest mortality in the very old and the very young. This has been a feature of the mortality pattern of all recorded outbreaks except that of 1918–1919, when there was a high mortality in young adults which has never been satisfactorily explained (Figure 12).

Epidemics of influenza appear to have occurred at various intervals from the 15th century to the 19th century. In 1840 following a number of years with no influenza, there was a pandemic of 'Russian flu', so called because of its supposed place of origin. This was followed by

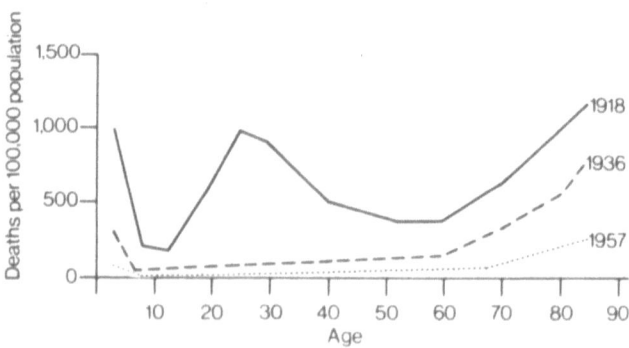

**Figure 12** Usual pattern of mortality from influenza in pandemic years compared with that of 1918 (deaths per 100 000 population)

pandemics of the 'Spanish flu' in 1918, which is estimated to have killed 20 million people, the 'Asian flu' of 1957 which circled the world within the year, the 'Hong Kong flu' of 1968, and the 1977 outbreak, which was a disease mainly affecting children.

The most widely accepted theory at present is that following genetic reassortment between two influenza A viruses, the resultant progeny possesses surface antigens of which the world population has had little or no previous experience. These major changes are represented as follows:

| 1930 | Puerto Rico (PR8) | A/H0N1 |
| 1946 | Fort Monmouth (FM1) | A/H1N1 |
| 1957 | Asian | A/H2N2 |
| 1968 | Hong Kong | A/H3N2 |
| 1977– | H3N2; still circulating | A/H1N1 |
| 1986 | ? | |

Antigenic shifts may be a survival mechanism of the virus. When a particular strain passes through a human population and more and more people become immune, only the mutants will survive in immune individuals. A population of mutant viruses will then gradually build up and give rise to a new strain. Why should this antibody 'drive' influence influenza and not other viruses? There is no evidence of viruses such as measles, mumps or rubella undergoing antigenic changes under the influence of antibody. Paradoxically, although influenza virus is a superficial type of infection with less contact with antibody-forming cells, it seems to undergo mutational changes more readily. But, furthermore, (1) there is no viraemia in influenza infections which would provide an opportunity for the antigen to stimulate as many antibody cells as possible throughout the body and (2) the short infectivity of the disease provides a shorter period of antigenic stimulation and the short incubation period of influenza (and other respiratory infections) reduces the time during which the body can mount a specific immune response to reinfection.

It is difficult to assess accurately the duration of immunity to influenza virus because it seems to vary with different strains and the degree of immunity has to be measured by natural challenge.

In contrast to influenza A virus, B and C viruses appear to have only one subtype and any antigenic change which occurs in them is very small. Influenza B, although apparently endemic, seems to spread

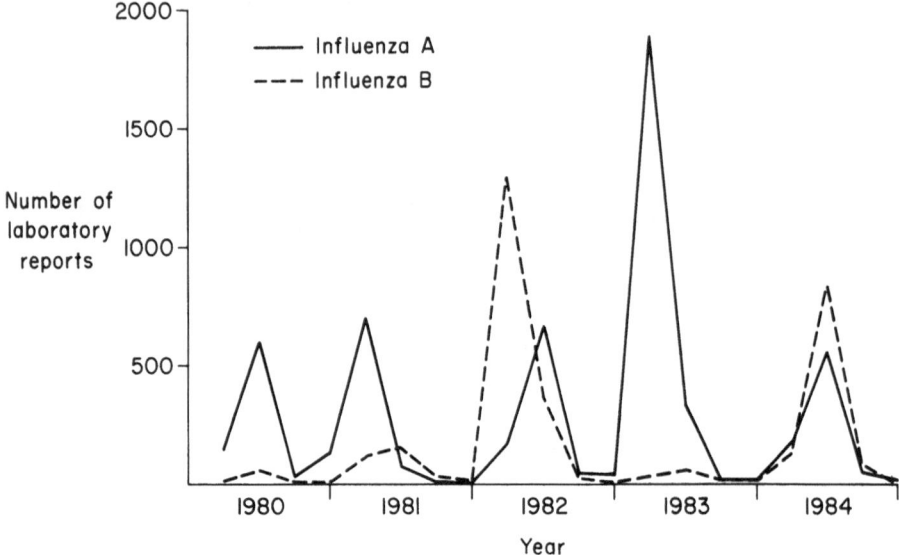

**Figure 13**   Recent outbreaks of influenza, England and Wales. (Prepared by CDSC)

poorly and produces only sporadic and local outbreaks every few years but not explosive pandemics. Influenza C only rarely produces outbreaks; however, it appears to circulate widely.

During the past few years the outbreaks of influenza have been relatively mild with both influenza A and B (Figure 13).

If the previous pattern of pandemics about every 10 or so years prevails, perhaps we can expect a pandemic in 1987. But prediction is a dangerous game and no one would have expected that two immunologically different A strains would have been running together over recent years.

## Morbidity

The annual number of days claimed for sickness benefit due to influenza in the UK in the past 20 years has varied from about 6 to 26 million, and the United States National Health Survey estimated that, with the advent of influenza A2 virus in 1957, during the 8 weeks from

29 September to 23 November there were 70 million new cases with 'bed disability' and a peak of 12 million in the week of 13 October. As well as much morbidity, influenza also produces considerable mortality, particularly in the elderly and those suffering from chronic disease. In England and Wales in a fairly 'good' winter, perhaps 3000–4000 old or debilitated individuals die of influenza. Nearly 70 000 deaths were attributed to influenza in the USA in 1957–1958.

## Control

With the exception of amantadine, slow progress has been made in controlling the infectivity of influenza with antiviral drugs. Amantadine is of some use in the prevention and treatment of influenza and has been recommended for high risk patients who cannot be or have not been immunized.

Theoretically, quarantine of infected individuals could control the source but this is not practicable with influenza. In a small island not dependent on world commerce, all visitors could be excluded in the face of a pandemic wave of a highly lethal strain, but otherwise any other control of the human source is at present impossible. If it is discovered that certain animals are reservoirs of influenza virus some animal control might be initiated. As far as breaking the chain of infection is concerned, in some countries, e.g. the USSR, the wearing of face masks has been recommended during epidemics. This could interrupt the person-to-person spread of droplets, but an individual who had successfully protected himself from infection during work or travel might quite readily pick up the virus at home from his family.

It is possible that, in general, children excrete larger quantities of viruses than adults and that they are the transmitters of infectious diseases *par excellence*. With influenza they may have had least experience with the viruses of the past and have no antibody to earlier related strains and little cell-mediated immunity. If this is so, it would seem sensible during outbreaks of influenza to try to reduce the contact between children and the elderly or the chronically sick. Influenza tends to have a higher mortality in the old and sick than in other susceptibles and flu (and other viruses) can precipitate an attack of bronchitis in those who suffer from that disease.

## Immunity to influenza

It would seem that antibodies to the haemagglutinin (H) and to a less extent to neuraminidase (N) play the most important part in protection. Since the H and N are constantly changing, the protective antibodies are of value for only a short time and immunity may only last for less than 1 year.

Evidence exists to suggest that an individual exposed to influenza virus will not only produce antibody to the infecting strain but will experience an anamnestic response of antibody to strains of the same group of viruses which had infected him in the past. The greatest response is to the most distant infection. This implies that influenza virus is an antigenic mosaic and suggests that the variations in H and N may be limited.

Although immunity to natural infection or experimental challenge is related to the possession of antibodies to the specific H and N of the challenge virus, presumably, other factors are involved in protection, e.g. cell-mediated immunity.

## Vaccines

The vaccines currently available in Western Europe and in North America are inactivated preparations of the current strains. They may be monovalent (e.g. H1N1 vaccine) but are usually multivalent (e.g. the vaccine for 1984/85 = A/Brazil/78 (H1N1), A/Bangkok/79 (H3N2) and B/Singapore/79 (H3N2)). The strains to be included in vaccines are reviewed annually by a WHO committee and changes are recommended as and when required to meet the challenges of antigenic 'drifts' and 'shifts'. In the preparation of influenza vaccines, the viruses are grown in the allantoic cavity of developing chick embryos and inactivated and purified. This constitutes a *whole virus* vaccine. A *split virus* vaccine is available which is prepared by disrupting the virus particles with detergents and partially purifying the disrupted particles by zonal ultracentrifugation. A third type of vaccine consists of purified haemagglutinin and neuraminidase. There is no adequate comparison of the comparative protective efficacy of the three available inactivated vaccines provided the current epidemic strains are included in the vaccine and there is good coverage of the exposed population: this type of influenza vaccine is claimed to have produced about a 60–70% protection. However, such protection is of limited duration, sometimes only about 4–6 months, although it may persist for up to 5 years following vaccination.

The problems of the efficacy of inactivated influenza vaccines relate to the observations that

(1) repeated 'drifts' may be summated over the years and markedly alter the antigenicity of any strain, so that a vaccine made to an earlier version of the same strain may be relatively ineffective and 'shifts' may take place so rapidly that the current circulating virus evades the protection provided by the vaccine;

(2) the protective antibodies elicited by the vaccine to the current or anticipated virus may be short lived.

At the present time adults and children of 13 years and older should require only one dose of vaccine for protection against the current strains. With a new pandemic strain, two doses of vaccine may be required at 4-week intervals. Younger children, because of their lack of experience with strains of virus related to the current strains, will certainly require two doses unless they have been previously or recently immunized with influenza vaccine.

The potency of influenza vaccine is measured in haemagglutination units and it is usually given by deep subcutaneous or intramuscular injection in a dose of 0.5 ml. (Efficiently maintained and expertly used jet injectors have been said to be satisfactory for administration of the vaccine.)

To facilitate the administration of inactivated vaccines, and in the hope of stimulating nasal antibody (IgA), trials of giving the vaccine intranasally have been carried out. However, these have not shown any obvious advantages in protection or antibody production.

Some have suggested that in order to produce durable protection, annual routine immunization is desirable, but in view of 'drifts' and 'shifts', I know of no good evidence to support this view. The available vaccines neither provide complete protection nor seem to retain their effectiveness when given annually but it is difficult to evaluate the vaccines presently available in the general population.

## Reactions

In the past, inactivated influenza vaccines produced redness at the site of injection, malaise, headache and fever and these occurred more frequently in children. These reactions appeared to be mainly due to non-viral protein, although influenza virus is itself toxic. The incidence of reactions has been greatly reduced in modern vaccines by the purification techniques now employed in their preparation. *Split* virus and *purified* haemagglutinin and neuraminidase vaccines cause fewer reactions and are recommended for children, in whom the dose should be smaller than the adult dose.

In a recent mass vaccination campaign in the USA in which about 50 million doses of swine influenza vaccine were administered, there was an excess frequency of Guillain–Barré syndrome (GBS) at the rate of about ten cases in 1 million persons vaccinated, which was five to six times higher than the comparable average in unvaccinated persons. This vaccine was withdrawn. Continued surveillance has not subsequently implicated influenza vaccines with an excess risk of GBS.

## Who should be immunized?

Although there was a *nationwide* immunization campaign in the USA to vaccinate against the H1N1 (swine) strain of virus, there seems to be no serious demand for wide-scale immunization against influenza in Europe. When people are immunized because an epidemic is anticipated and it fails to materialize, they are less enthusiastic about being vaccinated the following year when an unexpected epidemic may occur.

The serious nature of influenza does not seem to be generally appreciated and most people in Europe seem to be prepared to take the chance of not getting 'flu' during the winter and do not bother about vaccine. Yet in epidemic years, in addition to the excess mortality (i.e. when the number of deaths exceeds the norm for the given time and place), influenza causes the loss of millions of working days. (Of some interest in this respect was one controlled study which showed that immunization had saved about 14 working days per 100 employees. However, after the 'flu' outbreak those in the placebo group who had not been sick during the outbreak had the equivalent time off 'sick' – but not from influenza!)

The vaccines available at present are not recommended for routine use in an attempt to *control* epidemics but are said to be of value for 'high risk' groups. It is recommended that they should be vaccinated annually. They include the following.

(1) Patients with chronic pulmonary disease, e.g. bronchitis (who are especially vulnerable to influenza and in whom influenza can initiate an exacerbation). Also, those with emphysema, bronchiectasis, pulmonary tuberculosis, cystic fibrosis, chronic asthma and cardiovascular disease, especially those with mitral stenosis and with frank or incipient failure. Also included are patients with chronic diseases of the renal or nervous systems or with metabolic disorders.

(2) Elderly persons, particularly those living in institutions.

(3) Children living in institutions, including schools, where high attack rates can occur because of the facility of spread.

(4) Individuals such as doctors, nurses, ambulance men and other medical personnel who are at special risk of infection, and workers in other 'key' occupations.

There is some controversy about immunizing pregnant women and some experts do not consider this acceptable. There are conflicting reports on the possible incidence of congenital defects due to influenza virus: it does seem that in epidemic years there may be an excess fetal mortality. If a pregnant woman can be prevented from having influenza this outweighs any upset which might be caused by the injection of an inactivated virus vaccine.

## Contraindications

Vaccine should be used with caution in children because of the severity of reactions. They should be given appropriately smaller doses as indicated in the manufacturer's literature. The vaccine is contraindicated in individuals sensitive to egg products, poultry or feathers and in persons hypersensitive to polymyxin or neomycin.

## Future developments

One of the problems in preparing vaccines has been the adaptation of a new strain to grow in eggs, which delays its production. It is now possible to combine current strains with an old well-established high-growth laboratory strain and to produce a high-yield virus with the antigenic properties of the new strain. This can make vaccine production with a new strain possible in a few weeks, rather than months of adaptation of a new strain to produce a sufficient titre of virus. This recombination technique has made it possible to prepare viruses with the neuraminidase of one strain and the haemagglutinin of another and it is possible to swop virulence and other properties. It has been proposed that a 'library' of influenza viruses could be prepared which might contain the expected virus of the next epidemic. As soon as a new epidemic strain had been spotted and identified by one of the laboratories of the WHO surveillance network, a vaccine could be immediately manufactured.

With only a limited number of antigens – which seems a reasonable hypothesis because nature seldom has an infinite number of species or subspecies in any genus – it might be possible to make a vaccine containing all possible antigens.

## Live virus vaccines

Live virus influenza vaccines have been most intensely tested in the USSR but the methods of controlling many of the studies have been unsatisfactory. Massive immunization by aerosol vaccines in some cities in the USSR and also in Yugoslavia does not seem to have influenced epidemics to any great extent. Reactions in children to live influenza virus vaccines were considerably greater than in adults but vaccination by the intranasal route was said to have reduced these. The main problem was to attentuate the virus so that it would infect and immunize but not produce any disease. Over-attenuated strains which have produced no illness have not stimulated an adequate antibody response.

Theoretically, a live virus vaccine could be prepared in the face of an epidemic by mating the new virus with an avirulent well-adapted laboratory strain to produce an avirulent hybrid with the new antigens. A few thousand eggs could rapidly provide enough vaccine for millions of people and prevent many deaths in the face of a virulent epidemic. However, there are problems of safety testing and of the stability of such a virus vaccine when it replicates in man. Its potential for spread and mutation to virulence are unknown properties; however, recent studies of a cold-adapted reassortment influenza virus vaccine given intranasally against experimental challenge with homologous wild-type virus not only produced complete protection as compared with a 71% protection provided by inactivated vaccine, but also showed a great reduction in virus shedding, which suggests that it might more effectively limit transmission than could be achieved with inactivated vaccine.

# VIRAL HEPATITIS

Viral hepatitis may be caused by hepatitis A virus (HAV), hepatitis B virus (HBV) non-A,non-B viruses and the δ agent which is a satellite virus of HBV and which potentiates the hepatitis.

The non-A,non-B viruses are now frequently associated with post-transfusion hepatitis and are important causes of heaptitis in sub-tropical and tropical countries. The δ agent is antigenically related to hepatitis B virus from which it borrows its outer surface membrane; antibody to HBV will protect against it.

## Hepatitis A virus

Hepatitis A virus (HAV) causes infective jaundice. It is a member of the picornavirus group to which poliovirus also belongs. It may be grown in tissue culture and there is only one immunological type of the virus.

## The disease

The incubation period ranges from 15 to 50 days (mean = 30). The onset of jaundice is usually preceded by a prodromal period lasting for about 2 weeks with malaise, anorexia and often gastrointestinal symptoms with upper abdominal pain. The virus multiplies in the alimentary tract and the highest titres of virus occur before the onset of jaundice, which may last for a few weeks; complete recovery is usual. Anicteric cases may occur and the infection in children is often subclinical. HAV infection is not associated with the development of chronic liver disease and no virus carrier state has been identified.

A subclinical or a clinical infection of HAV gives lifelong immunity.

Serological tests of anti-HAV IgG are available which can identify individuals who are susceptible or immune to infection with the virus. HAV IgM develops before the onset of jaundice and while the anti-HAV IgM test is suitable for the diagnosis of an acute infection or recent infection, the levels of antibody may have reached a peak at the time of onset of jaundice and further rise in titre may not be significant.

## Epidemiology

Like poliomyelitis, the virus is spread by the faecal–oral route from a clinical or sub-clinical case by person-to-person contact. Food and water contaminated with faeces is an important source of infection, but it may also be transmitted by blood taken during the acute viraemic stage of the infection and by sexual intercourse. The maximum excretion of faecal virus occurs during the latter part of the incubation period (and before the onset of jaundice) at which time the patient is most infectious.

The number of cases of 'infective jaundice' (HAV infections) in England and Wales notified since 1969 are shown in Figure 14. During this period quite a remarkable change has taken place in the proportion of notification in the various age groups, as shown in Figure 15.

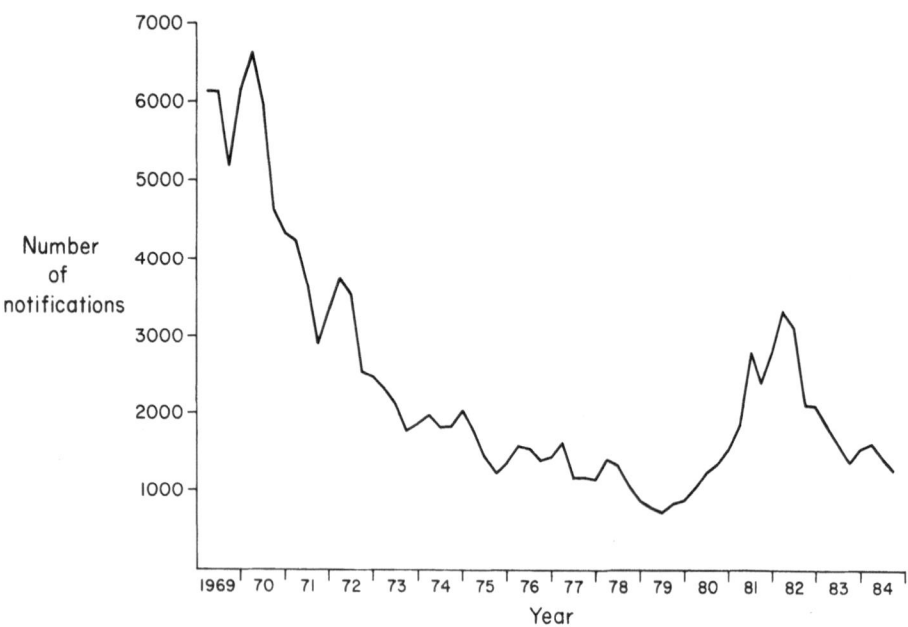

Source: Office of Population Censuses and Surveys

**Figure 14**   Infective jaundice. Corrected quarterly notifications, 1969–83. (Prepared by CDSC)

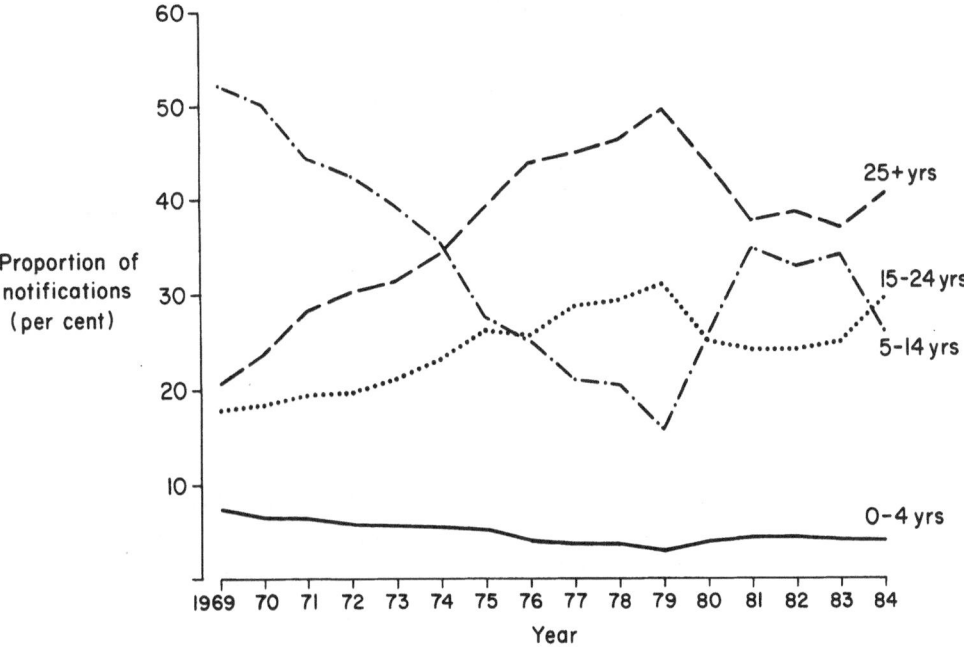

Source: Office of Population Censuses and Surveys

**Figure 15** Infective jaundice. Notifications in age groups, 1969–83, England and Wales. (Prepared by CDSC)

While in the late 1960s the disease was essentially an illness of schoolchildren, the highest proportion of notifications is now in the 25-year-and-older age group. Infective hepatitis is more frequent in countries with poor hygiene and visitors to these countries are at increased risk of infection, because of the free circulation of the virus in the community. It is possible that some of the changes in the age distribution are a reflection of overseas travels.

## Prevention

Control of HAV infection depends on personal and community hygiene (see Typhoid, page 146). Several studies are under way to develop a suitable vaccine, but meanwhile temporary protection may be obtained with normal human immunoglobulin (see page 180) which, of course, is not required for those individuals who have anti-HAV antibodies in their sera.

## Hepatitis B virus

Hepatitis B virus (HBV) infection, previously called 'serum hepatitis', is caused by a virus of the hepadnavirus group. The virus infects only primates and has not yet been grown in tissue cultures.

While infective hepatitis (infective jaundice, HAV) is a notifiable disease, information on the prevalence of HBV comes from laboratory reports. While laboratory reports of HAV correlate well with notifications, it is probable that the number of laboratory reports of HBV cases (Figure 16) represents the near total number of cases which occur.

## The virus

HBV has three major antigens known as the surface ($HB_sAg$), core ($HB_cAg$) and $HB_eAg$ antigens. It also possesses a DNA polymerase, and the presence of DNA polymerase activity and $HB_eAg$ in the blood

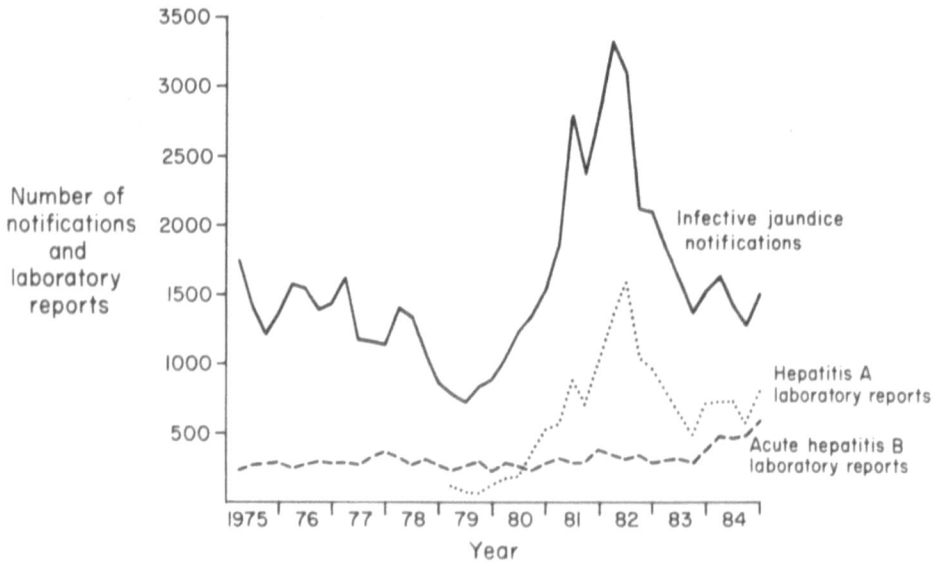

Source: Office of Population Censuses and Surveys and Communicable Disease Surveillance Centre

**Figure 16** Hepatitis. Quarterly notifications and laboratory reports, 1975–84, England and Wales. ———— = notifications of infective jaundice; ····· = laboratory reports hepatitis A; – – – – = laboratory reports hepatitis B. (Prepared by CDSC)

are indicative of high levels of circulating virus and of infectivity. The disease is prevented by an inactivated virus vaccine and because screening of patients who may require to be vaccinated is often done, it is necessary to be able to interpret the significance of the presence of the various viral antigens and their antibodies (Table 18).

**Table 18** Patterns of HBV serological markers demonstrated by specific radioimmune assays

| | Serological reactivity | | | |
|---|---|---|---|---|
| | | | Anti-HB$_c$ | |
| Diagnosis | HB$_s$Ag | Anti-HB$_s$ | IgG | IgM |
| Susceptible | – | – | – | – |
| Infection | | | | |
| Acute infection – early, or | | | | |
| late incubation period | + | – | – | – |
| Acute hepatitis | + | – | + | + |
| Chronic carrier | + | – | + | (+) |
| or rarely | – | – | + + | (+) |
| Immune | | | | |
| Recent acute or subclinical | – | + | + | – |
| infection, or | – | – | + + | (+) |
| Long past infection, or | – | + | – | – |
| | – | – | + | – |
| Following immunization | – | + | – | – |

## The disease

The incubation period ranges from 50 to 180 days (mean = 60–90). The clinical features of the disease are similar to, but much more severe than, those of type A hepatitis, but the majority of persons (50–60%) exposed to the virus experience a subclinical and asymptomatic infection. HB$_s$Ag is detectable in the sera of some of these individuals for only a brief period of time and they develop anti-HB$_s$, anti-HB$_c$ and rarely anti-HB$_e$. About 50% of infected individuals develop acute hepatitis with jaundice. In these patients anti-HB$_s$ arises during convalescence and is a marker of recovery and of immunity (it would also be indicative of immunization). About 5–10% of infected persons develop a chronic carrier state with a period of acute, sub-acute or chronic hepatitis followed in some by an asymptomatic carrier state with the disappearance of $HB_eAg$ and the appearance of anti-$HB_e$ but with the persistence of $HB_sAg$. Some of these carriers have chronic active or inactive cirrhosis of the liver and it is during this stage that hepatocellular carcinoma is likely to develop. It has been shown that the viral DNA of HBV becomes integrated into the tumour cells.

## Epidemiology

Infection normally occurs through the skin or mucosal surfaces and, as noted, HBV is usually transmitted from person to person by blood, which has the highest concentrations of HBV, but it may also be trans-mitted via the semen or saliva of carriers although probably less efficiently. HBV DNA is also found in urine. Transmission by trans-fusion of blood and blood products is now very rare in the UK because all these products are screened for HBV. As noted, the majority of cases of hepatitis following transfusion nowadays seem to be due to non-A,non-B viruses. (However, the onset of jaundice within 6 months of a transfusion of blood should raise the possibility of HBV infection).

There are said to be 200 million carriers of hepatitis B virus in the world (i.e. about 5% of the total world population). The vast majority live in South-east Asia and the Western Pacific countries. About 90% of infants born to mothers with high levels of circulating virus ($HB_eAg$ positive) may become carriers. Although hepatitis B acquired at birth seldom does any obvious harm in early life it is associated with serious liver disease in later years. This indicates the magnitude of the problem and of liver carcinoma of which HBV is an aetiological factor.

In warm climates infection occurs at all ages but in temperate climates the infection is rare in babies and in normal children and the majority of cases occur in young adults.

In the UK the number of overt cases identified annually is about 1000 and it is estimated that in Britain among the 50 000–60 000 infants born each year to non-white women about 400 could become per-sistent HBV carriers. In the USA there are said to be 200 000 new infections each year yielding 20 000 new carriers of the virus. While HBV is relatively uncommon in the indigenous population of northern

Europe, as would be expected it is frequent among immigrants from countries of high endemicity who are more likely to be carriers than e.g. the predominant white ethnic group of the British Isles.

There are essentially three groups who are most frequently infected in the UK;

(1) Involuntary groups:

    (a) The involuntary group of post-transfusion patients and those receiving blood products (immunoglobulins are not involved), e.g. haemophiliacs and patients in dialysis or oncology units; both are now rare as a result of screening;

    (b) Inmates of homes for mental handicap patients (this frequency may be related to their immunodeficiency);

    (c) The family or household contacts of HBV carriers.

(2) The occupational group of health workers in contact with HBV patients, carriers, or their blood.

(3) The lifestyle group including:

    (a) Homosexually active males (perhaps females are protected from invasion by the stratified epithelium of the vagina compared with the readily traumatized columnar epithelium of the rectum);

    (b) Drug addicts using syringes (Figure 17);

    (c) Tattooed individuals and those receiving acupuncture (which could play a part in the very high rates in China).

## Vaccines

The presently available vaccine consists of purified formalin-inactivated $HB_sAg$, prepared from the plasma of human carriers. It has been shown to be free from the virus of acquired immunodeficiency syndrome (AIDS) and should protect against the $\delta$ agent which is antigenically identical to hepatitis B virus. The vaccine is given in three intramuscular doses in alum adjuvant. The second and third doses should be given at 1 and 6 month intervals. Each dose for adults should contain $20\,\mu g$ $HB_sAg$ protein, $10\,\mu g$ for infants and children less than 10 years of age and $40\,\mu g$ for immunocompromised patients.

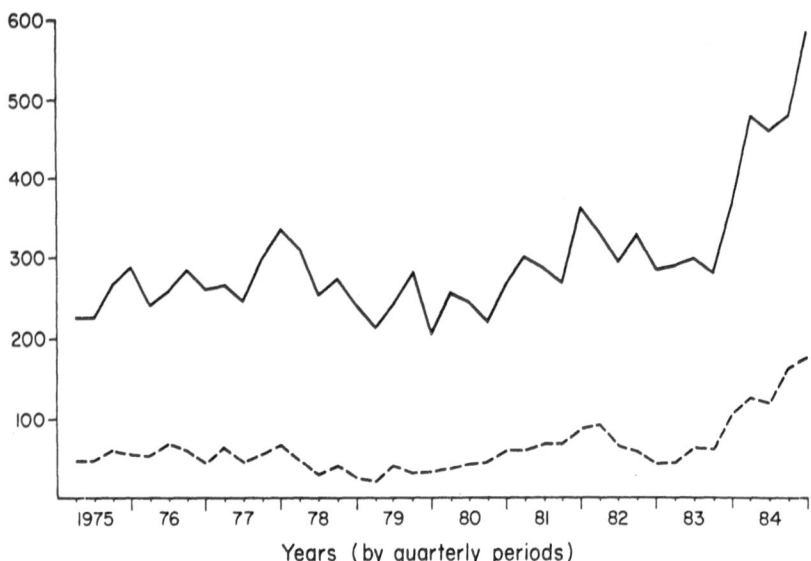

**Figure 17** Laboratory reports of acute HBV hepatitis with $HB_sAg$ (————) and number of cases with a known history of drug abuse (– – – – –), 1975-84, England and Wales - reports from Ireland are also included. (Prepared by CDSC)

The need for booster doses is not yet known. In babies at high risk of hepatitis B infection (born to $HB_sAg$ positive mothers or living with chronic $HB_sAg$ carriers), three doses of vaccine must be used and the first dose must be given at birth in combination with HBIg. (In children of more than 1 year of age a two-dose regimen may be considered.) The vaccine should be given into the arm rather than the buttock, in which there is a lower response rate (see p. 00).

The vaccine should be stored at 2-8°C but not frozen, as freezing destroys the potency of the vaccine and has been responsible for a drop in vaccine effectiveness from 90% to 85%.

About 95% of normal immunized persons develop anti-$HB_s$ after a course of vaccine which appears to afford protection against infection for at least 5 years.

The plasma vaccine, although highly effective, is very expensive (£63.50 for a full course, at the time of writing) and the extent of the viral hepatitis problem throughout the world has led to attempts to produce other vaccines using recombinant DNA technology. One of these is a recombinant yeast vaccine in which $HB_sAg$ was introduced into *Escherichia coli* and then into baker's yeast from which the antigen is released by homogenization. This yeast recombinant vaccine is now undergoing human trials. Another approach has been to develop synthetic vaccines which will certainly be the vaccines of the future.

## Who should be immunized?

At the present time, those at high risk of infection with HBV should be selectively immunized. It is debatable whether potential vaccinees should be screened for antibody prior to being given the vaccine. Screening for anti-HB$_s$ will detect most people who do not need immunization because they have had a natural infection, but 10% of people who *have* been infected in the past will not produce anti-HB$_s$, and anti-HB$_c$ is a more reliable marker. The decision to screen or not to screen depends on the epidemiological situation and on the cost of the vaccine and of its delivery, on the cost of screening and on the anticipated number of susceptibles in the group (as evidenced by a pilot serological study).

The first group to be considered for immunization are *health care personnel* and others directly involved in (1) the care of patients over a period of time where there is a known high incidence of HBV, (2) the care of patients in units where known carriers are treated, (3) work with blood and blood products – such as blood bank staff and laboratory workers exposed to increased risk of infection from infected material.

The second group to which the vaccine should be given are (1) patients on entry to residential institutes for the mentally handicapped where there is a known high risk, (2) specified renal dialysis patients and (3) specified spouses and other sexual partners and household contacts of HBV carriers, depending on their antibody status.

The third group are the high risk 'lifestyle' group which includes male homosexuals, drug abusers and also prisoners. Decisions to routinely immunize persons in this group will usually be made on cost-effective analysis and as far as the UK is concerned it would seem that there is a clear case to offer HBV vaccine to male homosexuals.

## *Immunization of infants*

Infants born to HB$_s$Ag positive women should receive specific HBV immune globulin (see page 183) but they should also receive vaccine (see above).

The above recommendations may change with the accumulation of more data.

## Emergency immunization

If the individual to be considered for emergency therapy is known to be susceptible to infection with HBV, then following a known single exposure to a *known* positive hepatitis B source, either by needle, by laboratory accident or by sexual contact, one dose of HBIG (0.06 ml/kg) should be given as soon as possible after exposure and at the same time the first dose of a course of vaccine injected at a different site. If the source of the infection is not known, then preferably a dose of HBIG should be given and the decision whether or not to immunize will depend on the results of tests for the HBV antigens which must be made available within a few days.

## Adverse reactions

All the evidence indicates that HBV vaccine is both safe and effective and that any side-effects are minimal. No long term reactions have been observed.

## Passive Immunization

This is discussed in Chapter 13.

## MUMPS

Mumps is caused by a paramyxovirus which is readily cultivated in embryonated eggs and in tissue cultures. It may be prevented by an attenuated virus vaccine. This vaccine has been combined with measles and rubella vaccines (MMR) and is used for routine immunization of children in some countries (see page 90). In the UK and in many other countries mumps vaccine is employed selectively.

## The disease

The symptoms and signs of mumps are swelling of the parotid gland and sometimes also the submandibular glands with or without malaise, fever, trismus and pain near the angle of the jaw. Parotitis seems to be a less frequent manifestation of mumps in summer than in winter.

In addition to infection of the salivary glands, other organs such as the c.n.s., testes, ovary, pancreas etc. may be involved. This may occur without parotitis – at the same time as, before or after parotitis. With the exception of involvement of the c.n.s. and testes, symptoms of infection of organs other than the salivary glands are rare.

Infection of the meninges may be fairly common but is usually symptomless. It may give rise to headache and bradycardia. Sometimes, there may be signs and symptoms of aseptic meningitis (ASM) or meningoencephalitis, and mumps virus is one of the commonest viral causes of ASM. Complete recovery with no sequelae is usual but a number of patients may have a long convalescence with 'nervousness', occasional headache and muscle weakness. Nerve deafness is a rare complication.

Unilateral or bilateral orchitis is said to occur in about 20% of post-pubertal clinical infections. Even bilateral mumps orchitis very rarely leads to sterility.

## Epidemiology

Mumps is spread by direct person-to-person contact by droplets from the upper respiratory passages, and man is the only known reservoir of the virus. The disease is endemic in urban communities and is commoner in the winter months when upper respiratory tract infections are more frequent.

In the past, there seemed to be peaks of infections every 7–8 years but it appears from data from the Royal College of General Practitioners that the disease is now peaking at 2–3-year intervals. At the same time it appears that the epidemiological features of mumps infections are changing from those of an epidemic disease in young adults and older children to a more endemic disease in younger children with the highest attack rates in children between 5 and 9 years of age, when complications are less frequent. The disease is more common in males than in females.

In the UK and in North America about 30–40% of adults who do not recall having had mumps will have had subclinical infections as evidenced by the presence of antibody. An attack of mumps results in lifelong immunity and in some Western countries it appears from serological surveys that more than 90% of adults are immune.

## Vaccine

In 1968 a live attenuated mumps virus (the Jeryl Lynn strain, named after the child from whom it was isolated) was licensed in the United States. This 'wild' virus was attenuated by culture in embryonated hens' eggs and chick-embryo tissue culture. Vaccines prepared from that strain are said to be about 95% effective. This is measured by the development of detectable antibody, following the subcutaneous injection of approximately 5000 $TCID_{50}$ in 0.5 ml. The levels of neutralizing antibody which develop are about one fifth of the levels found after natural infection; demonstrable antibody persists for at least 6 years after vaccination and might be expected to be durable.

## Who should be immunized?

In the USA it is said that at least half of the population are ill with mumps during their lifetime and that it accounts for considerable school absenteeism and hospitalization of 1% of cases! A substantial case has been made in that country and in Scandinavia for the intro-duction of mumps vaccine in the combined mumps/measles/rubella (MMR) vaccine which should inhibit any adverse effect of adding another vaccine to routine immunization programmes.

In the UK there is little demand for vaccination against mumps, and at present there seems no reason for its routine introduction for the immunization of all children. Mumps vaccine should certainly not be allowed to take priority over more essential community immunization programmes. There may be a place for its selective use in children reaching puberty who have not had mumps. Nearly half of such children will have had a subclinical infection, and it is now relatively simple, using radial haemolysis analysis, to identify susceptible children who require immunization. The mumps skin test is not a reliable indicator of immunity.

Mumps vaccine should be recommended for susceptible adults living in closed and isolated communities and installations and for children in residential homes, basically to reduce the nuisance of an outbreak of mumps. If screening and immunization of susceptibles is not employed in these situations, vaccine might be introduced on the diagnosis of the first case.

## Contraindications

Mumps vaccines have the same general contraindications as other live virus vaccines (see pages 17–18). It is also contraindicated in neomycin-sensitive individuals. It should not be given to pregnant women since the possible effects on fetal development are not known. It is not recommended in children less than 1 year old.

Experience of the use of this vaccine is limited and the literature accompanying the vaccine should be consulted.

# MENINGOCOCCAL MENINGITIS

Meningococcal meningitis is caused by Gram-negative diplococci of the *Neisseria* genus found only in human beings. They have polysaccharide capsules which determine their classification into eight subgroups.

The most extensive studies of the distribution of the various groups have been made in the USA and, in frequency, the main ones causing disease there and in other countries appear to be A, B and C, Y and W135. The meningococci are very frequent inhabitants of the nasopharynx and worldwide in distribution.

## Disease and epidemiology

The meningococcus is the commonest of all causes of bacterial meningitis. In most countries outbreaks are sporadic and are usually confined to closed communities, but epidemics have been reported from all parts of the world with a particular preponderance in the 'cerebrospinal fever belt' which lies between 4° and 16°N, from the Atlantic to the Red Sea. In the Sudan epidemics of 10 000–100 000 cases have occurred about every 10 years with attack rates up to five per 1000 population. A, B and C serogroups have been found in most outbreaks, and A epidemics have been the most severe – in some of which the highest incidence has, for some reason, been in older children.

Since most individuals become carriers of meningococci at one time or another, the majority of the population except small children become immune and the highest incidence of the disease is usually in the first 2 years of life.

## Vaccines

Bivalent A–C vaccines and quadrivalent (A, C, Y, W135) vaccines are commercially available for the prevention of meningococcal disease. The vaccines contain 50 mg of the specific polysaccharides per dose and are given by subcutaneous injection. The serogroup A vaccine has a clinical efficacy for at least 1 year with protection being achieved 1–2 weeks following immunization. The vaccines are relatively ineffective in very young children who are most commonly affected.

## Who should be vaccinated

Routine vaccination is not indicated. The control of epidemics with vaccines requires early identification of the serogroup involved and obviously, the vaccine to be used must contain that type (preferably as a monovalent vaccine). The strategy employed will depend on the epidemiological situation.

Meningococcal vaccine might be used selectively to immunize high risk individuals (e.g. household contacts of a case) as a supplement to chemotherapy.

Travellers to any country where an epidemic is occurring should be vaccinated with the quadrivalent vaccine.

## PNEUMOCOCCAL INFECTIONS

*Streptococcus pneumoniae* (the pneumococcus) is a characteristically lancet-shaped diplococcus which grows in pairs. Virulent pneumococci have polysaccharide capsules of which there are 83 different serotypes.

## The disease

The common diseases caused by pneumococci are pneumonia, meningitis and pneumococcal bacteraemia which have their highest attack rates in the very young and in the elderly, and otitis media in children.

Although improved social conditions and antibiotics have decreased the mortality and morbidity caused by the pneumococcus it is very difficult to get accurate data on the incidence of the various diseases which it causes or to evaluate the efficacy of pneumococcal vaccines by conventional trials. It seems that certain of the types of pneumococci are a more frequent cause of the diseases in most parts of the world (although there are differences) which makes it possible to construct vaccines with polysaccharides to the most frequently occurring pneumococcal types.

Each of the polysaccharides can elicit a specific serological response which is associated with immunity to pneumococcal infection with the type in question. Immunity appears to be durable for at least 5 years in adults but not in children.

## Vaccines

Vaccines have been made with varying compositions of the most frequent serotypes.

## Who should be vaccinated?

These vaccines are not effective in children under 2 years of age.

Routine immunization of healthy adults is not recommended but, based on studies in miners in South Africa and natives of Papua New Guinea, there may be a place for the selective use of pneumococcal vaccines in defined populations in certain areas. It does not seem to have been effective in homes for the elderly, although some studies have shown that compared with treatment it may be cost-effective in persons of 65 years and over.

Various high risk groups have been defined where pneumococcal infection carries a high risk. These include sickle cell disease which unfortunately has the highest risk in the age group where the vaccine is least effective. There are conflicting reports on the efficacy of the vaccine in Hodgkin's disease and in splenectomized patients. It does not appear to be of any value in preventing recurrent otitis media. While primary immunization is generally free of serious adverse reactions, reinjection of the vaccine may give rise to severe local reactions of the Arthus type with fever in about 50% of those vaccinated.

Widespread use of pneumococcal vaccines in high risk groups must await further evidence of its efficacy. Meanwhile, because of the adverse effects which may follow reinjection of pneumococcal vaccines, agreement should be reached on a single pneumococcal vaccine formulation.

## Contraindications

The vaccine is contraindicated in children under 2 years of age and in pregnancy and should be used with caution in cardiovascular and respiratory diseases.

## ANTHRAX

Anthrax is caused by an anaerobic spore-bearing bacillus. The spores may remain viable for many years and have even been found in the so-called 'virgin' lands of Siberia. Anthrax is primarily a disease of sheep, cattle and horses which become infected by ingesting or inhaling the spores. After germination, the bacilli spread from the lymphatics into the blood stream where they multiply extensively.

## The disease

In humans anthrax gives rise to a cutaneous lesion which first appears as a papule and develops into a pustule which rarely contains pus (the so-called 'malignant pustule'), proceeding to a necrotic ulcer giving rise to a black eschar. The infection may disseminate and give rise to a septicaemia. Inhalation of spores may give rise to 'wool sorter's disease', a primary pneumonia which is often rapidly fatal.

## Epidemiology

The disease is rare in the UK and USA. Essentially an occupational disease, it occurs in those exposed to infected hides and carcasses and to imported bonemeal, fishmeal and feeding stuffs.

The numbers of notifications and deaths in 5-year periods from 1960 are shown in Table 19.

revention depends on controlling anthrax in animals and by sterilizing imported hides, wool and hair. However, it is uneconomic to sterilize bonemeal, and those handling it – e.g. warehousemen and gardeners – should be advised to wear gloves when doing so.

**Table 19**  Annual reports of anthrax and deaths (corrected) to the Chief Medical Officer for England and Wales

| Year | 1960–4 | 1965–9 | 1970–4 | 1975–9 | 1980–4 |
|------|--------|--------|--------|--------|--------|
| Notifications | 42 | 48 | 21 | 15 | 2 |
| Deaths | 3 | 5 | 5 | 0 | 0 |

## Vaccines

A vaccine is available for anyone subject to heavy exposure. It consists of an extract of *B. anthracis* and is given in a course of four intramuscular injections, each of 0.5 ml. The first three injections are given at 3-weekly intervals and the fourth about 6 months later. Reinforcing doses should be given at about yearly intervals.

## Reactions

Reactions are usually only local at the site of injection and are rare.

## Contraindications

There are no specific contraindications.

# 11
# Vaccination for Travel

'Come to Carnival in Rio
Visit Sunny North Africa
Tour the Game Parks of Kenya
See the Taj Mahal by moonlight
And come home sick'

(B. G. Maegraith)

It is the duty of individuals travelling abroad to be aware of the measures they should take to protect themselves against the diseases prevalent in the countries to be visited or passed through. Their attention should be drawn to government pamphlets such as *Protect your Health Abroad* (DHSS) obtainable (gratis) from travel agents, local Social Security offices or the DHSS Pamphlet Unit, PO Box 21, Stanmore, Middx. HA7 1AY, and to *Health on Holiday and other Travels* – a family doctor booklet published by the British Medical Association, Tavistock Square, London WC1H 9JR and available from the BMA or from High Street chemists (60p). The US Department of Health Education and Welfare produces *Notice to Travellers*. All travel agents should have a copy of *Vaccination Certificate Requirements for International Travel and Health Advice to Travellers* (1984) with addenda (Geneva: WHO; London: HMSO; £4.80). Because of changes in health requirements the DHSS pamphlet is updated on PRESTEL. Intending travellers to countries outside Europe and North America should also seek information from the embassy or mission of the countries to be visited (although the information supplied by most of them is often of little value and out of date). Recently a computerized data base has been set up in the Bureau of Hygiene and Tropical Diseases (Keppel Street, London WC1E 7HT) by the Medical Advisory Service to Travellers Abroad and most information on health risks and immunization required for foreign travel may be obtained for a fee.

## Diseases requiring International Certificates

No country now requires an International Certificate of Vaccination against smallpox from any traveller but the health regulations of some require International Certificates of vaccination against cholera and yellow fever from travellers entering or leaving these countries.

# CHOLERA

Epidemic cholera is caused by comma-shaped bacteria called vibrios – the classic *Vibrio cholerae* and *V. eltor* biotypes each with Ogawa and Inaba serotypes. They infect humans through the ingestion of water contaminated with the faeces or vomitus of patients, with the faeces of 'carriers', or by contaminated food, and people with blood group O seem to be more susceptible. Having passed the stomach, where *V. cholerae* is readily inactivated by the gastric juice, it colonizes the small intestine and liberates an enterotoxin (choleragen) which causes a great increase in adenylate cyclase activity and cAMP concentration; this results in the outpouring of water and chloride and the inhibition of absorption of sodium in the small intestine with resultant diarrhoea – sometimes massive – up to 20 litres daily of 'rice water' stools – dehydration, acidosis and shock. No one need die of cholera if properly treated with vigorous replacement of the lost electrolytes and fluids by intravenous or oral therapy.

The presently available vaccines do not have any significant impact on the endemicity or epidemicity of the disease.

## History and epidemiology

It would seem that until the beginning of the last century cholera was confined to the continent of Asia and was not a serious pandemic disease. However, in 1817 an extensive outbreak in the Ganges delta spread throughout large parts of Asia and Africa during the next 6 years and then disappeared. Following this, other waves of infection have spread from India, and in the second and third pandemic, in the 19th century, the disease reached Britain, Canada and the USA which were infected by Irish immigrants. In the London outbreak in 1848–9 John Snow (of Broad Street pump fame) was able to show conclusively, by applying the scientific method to the study of an epidemic, that cholera was transmissible by faecal contamination of water.

Cholera disappeared from the UK at the end of the last century and from other countries which developed sewage disposal and water purification techniques. For many years cholera appears to have been confined to the edges of the Ganges and Brahmaputra rivers, then in 1961 the seventh pandemic arose, caused by a new biotype called el tor (after a quarantine station in Egypt). This pandemic started in the Indonesian Archipelago and spread throughout South-east Asia in 1963, to the India–Pakistan subcontinent in 1964, the Middle East in 1965-6 and to Eastern Europe, West and North Africa and to Spain in the 1970s, threatening much of the rest of Europe and the Americas (Figure 18). Nobody knows why the el tor pandemic was so widespread but it seems that there were many carriers or symptomless excretors and many more mild cases of diarrhoea than occurred with the classical biotype (*V. cholerae*) which began to be isolated in increasing frequency in Bangladesh in 1982 replacing the el tor biotype.

## Control

The extent of any outbreak following an importation will be governed by the standards of public and personal hygiene of the community. Control depends on maintaining levels of personal and community hygiene which will prevent faecal–oral spread of the vibrios. Vegetables which have been irrigated with sewage, or shellfish from sewage-infected water, are potent sources of infection. In many parts of the world it is wise to avoid drinking unsterilized water, eating from street stalls, or eating green salads or fruits which cannot be peeled or have not been immersed in water-sterilizing solution (see BMA's *Health on Holidays and other Travels*).

In recent years cholera has been imported to the UK on several occasions but did not spread. Further importations are likely to occur, so all physicians must be aware of the possibility of importation of cholera by tourists and migratory workers. Cholera should be suspected in patients with diarrhoea returning from an infected area. With the extensive movement of people nowadays, it has been suggested that in a few years *V. cholerae* might be as common as *Shigella sonnei* in schools and institutes in Western Europe. Hopefully, as in other pandemics of cholera, it will disappear.

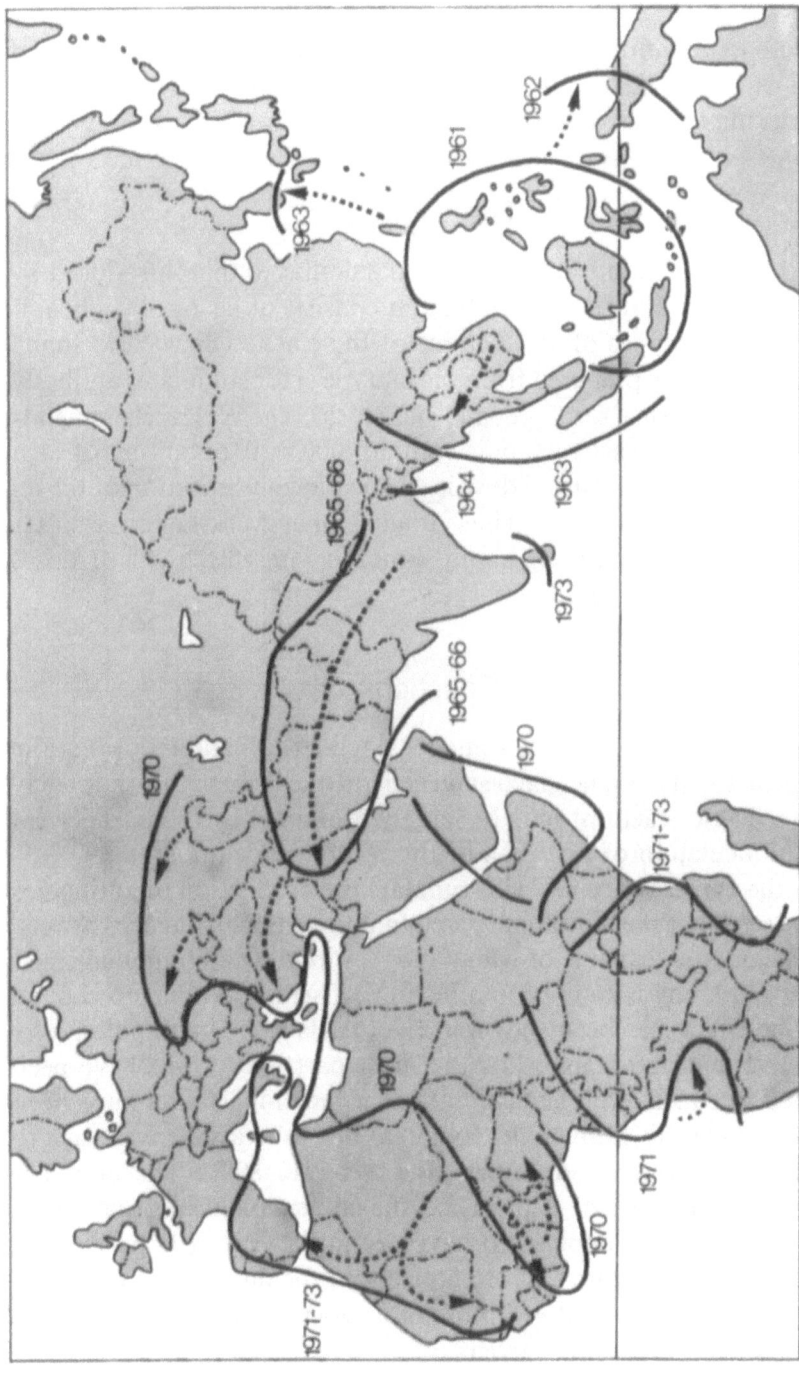

**Figure 18** Global spread of cholera, 1961–73 (WHO)

## Immunization

As noted, immunization plays no part in the control of outbreaks and should not be used in managing the contacts of imported cases nor for attempting to control the spread of infection.

## The vaccine

The vaccine available at present is very similar to that introduced by Kolle at the end of the last century. It consists of heat-killed phenol-preserved serotypes of *V. cholerae* of the classic Ogawa and Inaba strains. (Vaccine prepared from the biotype el tor stimulates antibody against the classical serotypes and vice versa.) The WHO recommends that each dose of vaccine should contain $4000 \times 10^6$ organisms of each serotype per ml. The usual dose is a subcutaneous injection of 0.5 ml followed by 1.0 ml of vaccine about 3 or 4 weeks later. Booster injections are required at about 6-month intervals: reduced doses should be given to children.

## Reactions

Occasionally, there may be some local tenderness and redness at the injection site. Fever, headache and general malaise and diarrhoea may occur. These reactions may be largely prevented by the intradermal (i.d.) inoculation of one fifth of the recommended dose.

While cholera vaccines will stimulate the production of antibodies in the serum, it must be appreciated that there is a difference between 'antigenic' (i.e. capable of stimulating antibody) and 'immunogenic' (i.e. stimulating immunity to infection). There is, so far, no cholera vaccine which has been shown in field trials to be immunologically effective and acceptable. For the most part these trials have been carried out in heavily endemic areas in individuals who have been immunologically primed. In some studies the vaccine was said to reduce the incidence of overt disease by 40–80%. The apparent efficacy of the vaccine depends on the epidemiological situation: in some, the vaccine appears to have produced very little protection. After a complete course of immunization, the duration of effectiveness may be only about 3–6 months. It does not prevent vaccinated persons from becoming carriers.

## International Certificates

International Cholera Vaccination Certificates are valid from 6 days after primary vaccination for a period of 6 months. On revaccination within 6 months a certificate is immediately valid for a further 6 months. At the present time it is agreed in International Health Regulations that cholera vaccination is no longer required for admission to most countries no matter where travellers come from. However, at the time of writing, Nigeria requires that travellers leaving Nigeria for a country where cholera vaccination is required will need a vaccination certificate. India's ruling is that travellers proceeding to countries that impose restrictions for arrivals from India or from a cholera infected area in India are required to possess a certificate.

A cholera vaccination certificate will not prevent the introduction of the disease into any country! In addition the requirement of such a certificate is in excess of the International Health Regulations for those countries that are bound by the Regulations.

## Recommendations for immunization

The risk of cholera is very small for travellers using the usual tourist routes and accommodation, but vaccine is recommended for people travelling by unusual routes in countries where cholera is endemic or epidemic.

Secondly, since some countries may still require an International Cholera Vaccination Certificate from travellers, in order to facilitate foreign travel to endemic countries, or for transit, a dose of 0.1 ml of cholera vaccine given intradermally should suffice to satisfy the regulations of those countries still requiring proof of cholera vaccination for entry or departure.

## The future

Efforts to produce an effective toxoid vaccine prepared from choleragen were not met with success, but the possibility of using a live vaccine consisting of a mutant that produced an immunizing fraction of choleragen has been tested in human volunteers and shows some promise.

# YELLOW FEVER

Yellow fever is caused by a group B arthropod-borne (Arbo) virus of the genus *Flavivirus*: it may be prevented by the 17D attenuated virus vaccine.

## The disease

The disease is characterized by a haemorrhagic diathesis with fever, haematemesis (the dreaded 'black vomit') and jaundice. It is endemic in areas in Central and South America and in Africa between 25°N. and 5°S. (including the Sudan, Ethiopia and countries of West, Central and East Africa) (Figure 19). The case fatality rate in non-indigenous individuals in outbreaks has varied from 10% to 30%. There is often a high attack rate in the indigenous population with many subclinical cases but a case fatality rate of less than 5%.

## History and epidemiology

Yellow fever was at one time the scourge of West Africa (the 'white man's grave') and of the Caribbean and during the summer, the disease would spread by sea routes from these areas to coastal towns of Europe and up the coast and along the navigable rivers of North America. At the beginning of this century Walter Reed and his colleagues working in Cuba discovered that the disease was transmitted by the black and white mosquito *Aedes aegypti* and, by controlling the breeding places of this highly domestic mosquito, General Gorgas eradicated yellow fever from the Caribbean in a few weeks and it was soon controlled in adjacent areas. However, although urban yellow fever is transmitted from man to man by *A. aegypti*, the reservoir of the virus is among monkeys of the central rain forests of South America and of Central Africa where the disease is transmitted from monkeys to man by mosquitoes. It is obviously impossible to control the monkey reservoir or the forest mosquitoes, and the disease is prevented in man by immunizing people living or working in or on the edges of forests and visitors to endemic zones. (The virus from the forest can reach urban centres in the blood of infected people and can then spread if there is inadequate control of *A. aegypti*.)

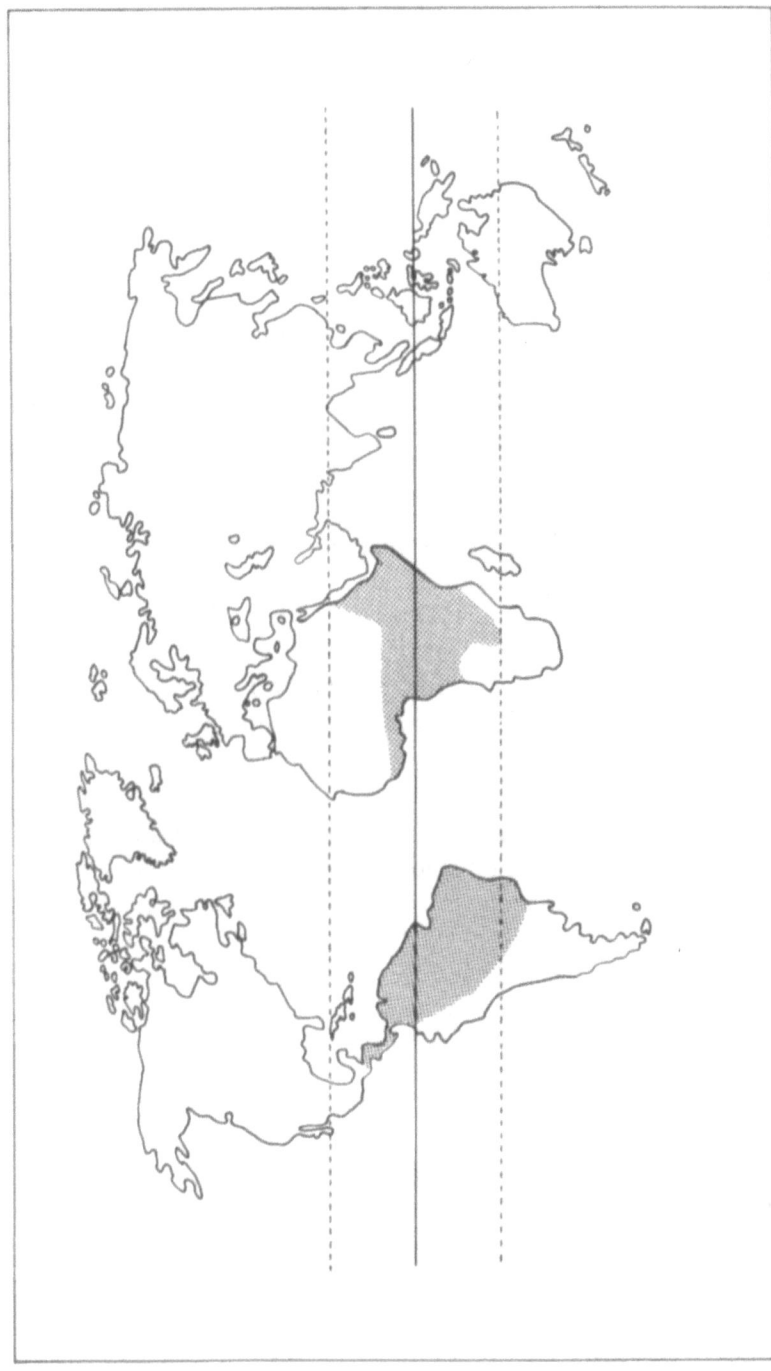

**Figure 19** Geographical distribution of endemic cases of yellow fever

In recent years the virus has reappeared in Southern Sudan (1940 and 1950), Panama (1949 and 1956), Ethiopia (1960–1), Peru (1969–70), Bolivia (1972), and Brazil (1973) and at the present time (1985) it is still present in all these countries except Panama and also in Brazil, Burkina Faso (formerly Upper Volta), Colombia, Ecuador, Gambia, Ghana, Nigeria and Zaire. The disease has never occurred in Asia or the Far East.

## Yellow fever vaccine

Yellow fever vaccine consists of an attenuated virus (17D) which was developed by repeatedly passing the virulent Asibi strain (recovered in West Africa from a patient of that name) intracerebrally in mice. The virus was further attenuated by passage in chick-embryo tissue culture. When this virus was injected into man, it replicated and circulated in the blood but produced no disease. For vaccine production on a large scale, the 17D virus is grown in the developing chick-embryo. Earlier batches of vaccine were most probably contaminated with avian leukosis virus, but the 17D strain is now propagated in eggs from leukosis-free flocks. Originally human serum was added as a stabilizing agent but this was stopped in 1942 when it led to an extensive outbreak of acute viral hepatitis amongst American troops in Northern Ireland, causing about 28 600 cases of jaundice among 2.5 million vaccinated soldiers, of whom 62 died.

The 17D vaccine used today is available only at designated centres. It is a freeze-dried preparation which is reconstituted in distilled water immediately before use. The dose is 0.5 ml given by deep subcutaneous injection and the vaccine may give lifelong immunity. The vaccine and the diluent should be stored at 4–8 °C.

## Contraindications

Unless specifically requested 17D vaccine should not be given to children under 9 months of age since it may give rise to encephalitis in young babies. Vaccine should not be given to individuals who are sensitive to eggs.

## Reactions

Very occasionally there may be a very mild local reaction at the site of injection or slight malaise about the seventh day after immunization.

## International Yellow Fever Certificates

These certificates are available after immunization at the relevant centre. They are valid 10 days after primary immunization and for 10 years thereafter and immediately valid for a further 10 years on revaccination. Certificates are required for travel to or through the endemic zones, but not for Asia or the Far East *unless* the traveller is arriving from a yellow fever area.

## Simultaneous immunization

Some interference between cholera and yellow fever immunization may occur if given at the same time, but it is not sufficient to influence schedules of immunization: if given together they should be injected at different sites.

As already noted, in order to sort out any reactions which might occur it is best to allow an interval of 3 weeks between the administration of two live virus vaccines.

When many immunizations are required, it is important to remember the time after immunization when the validity of an international certificate begins, in order to arrange suitable spacing of the vaccines.

## TYPHOID FEVER

Typhoid fever is caused by *Salmonella typhi* which is one of the more than 1000 species of salmonella. Their classification is based on their biochemical reactions and on three types of antigens – the flagellar (H), the O and the Vi antigens of the polysaccharides of the cell wall. Unlike the other *Salmonella* spp. it is exclusively a human pathogen.

## The disease

As in the case of *V. cholerae*, *S. typhi* enters by the mouth and having succeeded in passing the stomach barrier, unlike *V. cholera*, it is invasive and enters the lymphatics and multiplies in the lymph nodes of the intestine, spleen, bone marrow and liver and then multiplies in the gallbladder, which can produce a continuous source of reinfection of the intestines and a carrier state in about 2% of patients. After an incubation period of 10–14 days the symptoms of the clinical disease become apparent with the onset of bacteraemia. These consist of somewhat indefinite non-specific symptoms in the first week with fever and malaise often with constipation, followed by sustained fever, headache, abdominal pain and diarrhoea or constipation. Since typhoid fever has an incubation period of 10–14 days, it should always be suspected in a person with PUO of 3 or more days who has recently returned from travel in an endemic area.

## Epidemiology

Although *S. typhi* is a human pathogen it can multiply in food and in water in which it can survive for weeks or months. The source of contamination is usually a chronic carrier or a subclinical or clinical case. Typhoid is essentially a disease of developing countries, and outbreaks are rare in Northern Europe or in North America, but some will recall the outbreaks in Croydon (1937), Zermatt (1963) and Aberdeen (1964).

Lack of accurate diagnosis and reporting makes it impossible to enumerate the extent of typhoid infections throughout the world but in general the proportion of cases being reported in developed countries arising from foreign travel is increasing.

The total number of cases of typhoid fever in England and Wales in 1978–82 was 1092 as ascertained by the Communicable Disease Surveillance Centre and the rates of infection of UK travellers overseas is shown in Table 20.

Of these cases 134 (12%) were contracted in Britain presumably from a household chronic carrier or were in immigrants or visitors from the Indian subcontinent or other endemic area. 106 (10%) were contracted in Spain and the Mediterranean area, but the risk of a holidaymaker in these areas contracting typhoid fever is less than one per 100 000 visitors. Typhoid fever is predominantly a disease of children of school age and young adults; it is rarely reported in infants: the data from CDSC shows that of the cases contracted in Britain 26% were in preschool children, 12% in schoolchildren and 10% in adults.

**Table 20**  Typhoid fever: rates of infection in UK travellers overseas, 1978–84

| Year | Indian subcontinent No. of cases | Indian subcontinent Rate per 100 000 travellers | Mediterranean No. of cases | Mediterranean Rate per 100 000 travellers | Middle East No. of cases | Middle East Rate per 100 000 travellers | West Africa No. of cases | West Africa Rate per 100 000 travellers |
|---|---|---|---|---|---|---|---|---|
| 1978 | 168 | 128.2 | 52 | 0.7 | 11 | 5.7 | 7 | 18.0 |
| 1979 | 143 | 96.0 | 26 | 0.3 | 19 | 9.6 | 9 | 23.1 |
| 1980 | 156 | 99.4 | 20 | 0.2 | 8 | 3.7 | 11 | 24.4 |
| 1981 | 113 | 66.9 | 33 | 0.3 | 8 | 3.5 | 13 | 27.1 |
| 1982 | 98 | 45.4 | 17 | 0.1 | 3 | 1.4 | 24 | 55.8 |
| 1983 | 121 | * | 47 | 0.3 | * | * | 11 | 26 (prov.) |
| 1984 (prov.) | 101 | * | 6 | 0.03 | * | * | 13 | 27 (prov.) |

* Data not available

The prevention of typhoid is (1) by identifying the most important sources of infection, i.e. chronic carriers or subclinical cases, and excluding them from work where they are likely to transmit the bacteria to food or water and treating them; (2) by breaking the chain of infection by ensuring high standards of control of food and water and of sewage disposal and high standards of personal hygiene; (3) by immunization.

## Vaccines

Although inactivated typhoid vaccines had been available since the beginning of this century it was not until 1960 that a number of controlled field trials, sponsored by WHO, were carried out to ascertain their efficacy. These field trials were done in areas where typhoid is endemic (Yugoslavia, Guiana, Poland, USSR). Under these situations the vaccines tested gave a protection rate of 50–90% (depending on the vaccine used) when given in a course of two subcutaneous doses.

The duration of protection was variable, with some trials showing protection up to more than 90% during the first 3 years after immunization and 50–80% during the following 4 years. But these trials must not be applied to individuals living in the UK or other non-endemic countries, for many of the volunteers in the trials may have had subclinical infections before immunization and had their natural immunity primed by the vaccine. It is also possible that, following immunization, their vaccine-induced immunity was boosted by natural symptomless infections.

Challenge studies which have been done in volunteers not previously exposed to natural infections have shown that the protection afforded by the vaccine is dependent on the infective dose. It may be concluded that immunity can be more readily achieved against a water borne infection than one transmitted by food, where there would be a greater opportunity for multiplication of the bacilli.

The presently available vaccines usually consist of heat-killed, phenol-preserved S. *typhi* at a concentration of not less than 1000 million organisms per ml. The basic course recommended by the DHSS is two doses each of 0.5 ml (0.25 ml for children) given by deep subcutaneous or intramuscular injection at a 4–6-week interval, followed by a 0.5 ml reinforcing dose every 3 years. (If it is not possible to give the two doses of the basic course at a 4–6-week interval three doses at weekly intervals might be effective for those likely to be at high risk.) The second dose and the reinforcing dose may be given intradermally in a volume of 0.1 ml.

It is stated that for primary immunization 'one dose is almost as effective for a short period' as are two doses (DHSS). The evidence for this is contentious. In one field trial, where absenteeism resulted in children receiving only one dose of vaccine, they appeared to be as well protected as those receiving two (how similar are two groups one of which consisted of absentees?). In another field trial no protection could be demonstrated in children receiving only one dose. For adequate protection two doses appear to be required. I believe that a single primary dose of typhoid vaccine for visitors popping over to the Costa Brava is virtually useless unless they have some basic immunity to S. *typhi*. In any event it could not be effective (if at all) for about a fortnight after immunization and it provides a false sense of security about taking precautions against partaking of faecally contaminated food and drink.

Because of the adverse reactions associated with the subcutaneous injection of typhoid vaccine (see below) it would seem that the intradermal route should be used. The i.d. route has been used regularly and successfully in the British Army for about 25 years: one study showed that 0.1 ml of a vaccine containing $5 \times 10^9$ organisms per ml given i.d. gave responses similar to those of 0.5 ml of a vaccine containing $2.5 \times 10^9$ organisms given subcutaneously. Similar results have been provided by other studies. In general, as with other whole bacterial vaccines, the intradermal route has a fivefold adjuvant effect and 0.1 ml intradermally produces at least as strong an immune response (as measured by antibody production) as 0.5 ml given subcutaneously.

The correlation between the levels of antibodies against H, O and V antigens and protection against typhoid is under debate, but it would appear that the H antibody response is probably indicative of a protective vaccine. Although no field trials of the efficacy of administration of the basic course or boosting by the i.d. route have been done, since all the measurable laboratory responses are similar to those following subcutaneous or intramuscular injections, it is not unreasonable to assume a similar protective response.

## Reactions

Reactions after typhoid vaccine are common and include swelling, redness and pain at the injection site which usually occurs within a few hours of injection and lasts for about 2 days. General reactions including fever, malaise, headache and nausea are often present for 24–48 hours. Other rare complications of the cardiovascular, renal and central nervous system etc have been observed. Reactions are reduced when the intradermal route is employed. In the study in the British Army referred to, about 75% of the vaccinees had local reactions and 5-10% had general reactions following s.c. administration of the vaccine, compared with no general reactions and 1% with local reactions in the i.d. group. Again, in a similar recent study from Sweden 76% (25 of 33) of the group inoculated subcutaneously had 'severe' local reactions compared with 20% (nine of 45) of the i.d. group.

## Contraindications

Typhoid vaccine should not be given to babies under 1 year of age, among whom the disease is mild and of low incidence and reactions to the vaccine unpleasant.

Typhoid vaccine is not recommended in the face of an epidemic as it would have little or no effect and could interfere with the serological diagnosis of suspected cases.

It should not be given to individuals who are suffering from an illness.

## Recommendations

Immunization is *not* recommended for all holidaymakers going to Southern Europe or the Mediterranean areas where the risk of contracting typhoid is less than one case per 100 000 visitors (with more than 7 million visitors per year). I do not think that it should be routinely recommended for all travellers to the subtropics or the tropics. Certainly not for '*All* persons travelling abroad with the exception of those going to Canada, USA, Australia, New Zealand and Northern Europe' (DHSS).

It would seem wise to immunize intimate contacts of known typhoid carriers.

## The future

Typhoid immunization is a poor substitute for pure water and uncontaminated food but, because parenteral vaccines are not always highly effective and have undesirable side-effects, the search for a better vaccine continues. A safe and effective oral vaccine made from the *S. typhi* strain Ty21a which is a stable double mutant of the wild type Ty2 strain is now available and has been subjected to field trials with satisfactory results. This vaccine is given in a gelatin capsule with bicarbonate in order to facilitate the passage of the Ty21a bacteria through the stomach. With modern genetic techniques it should be possible to construct *S. typhi* 21a strains which could protect against other similar intestinal pathogenic bacteria at the same time as immunizing against typhoid fever.

## POLIOMYELITIS

Travellers to areas or countries where poliomyelitis is endemic or epidemic should be offered a reinforcing dose of OPV or IPV (see Chapter 6). In general, OPV is at present the vaccine of choice for supplementary doses of vaccine for travellers who have completed their primary courses of immunization. For those under 18 years of age, OPV vaccine may be given for primary and booster doses but IPV is the vaccine of choice for persons of 18 years of age and older who have not completed a primary course. For unimmunized persons who are departing for an endemic or epidemic country in less than 4 weeks, one dose of OPV is recommended and they should complete the course of immunization on return home.

## TICKBORNE ENCEPHALITIS

This disease is also known as central European encephalitis, Russian spring–summer encephalitis, Far Eastern encephalitis and diphasic milk fever. It is caused by a group B arbovirus of the flavivirus group which includes viruses which cause not only encephalitis but also haemorrhagic fever (e.g. Omsk haemorrhagic fever).

The disease usually occurs in the spring and summer when the vectors *Ixodes persulcatus* and *I. ricinus* are active in forested areas. Animals are also infected and the virus may be transmitted to man by drinking milk or consuming dairy products from infected cows or goats (diphasic milk fever).

Many infections are asymptomatic but they may result in encephalitis and a rapidly progressive fatal bulbar paralysis.

### Prevention

Prevention consists of avoiding tick-infested areas and using insect repellents containing DET (diethyltoluamide).

A vaccine is available for those whose work or leisure activities involve walking or camping in forested areas in Eastern Europe. Stocks of this vaccine are held in the UK by Immuno Limited, Dunton Green, Kent. It is recommended that for primary immunization two doses should be given 4–6 weeks apart and a reinforcing dose 12 months later should be given to those with continuing exposure to tick bites.

## JAPANESE ENCEPHALITIS

Japanese B encephalitis occurs in epidemics during the summer months particularly in the rainy season, in parts of India, Bangladesh, Korea, parts of China and the eastern part of the USSR.

The disease is caused by a group B arbovirus of the flavivirus group which is transmitted from domestic animals and birds to man by several species of mosquitoes.

The risk is minimal to short term travellers following normal routes and urban centres, but those who will be *resident* in an infected area should certainly consider immunization.

## Prevention

Prevention depends on taking all precautions against being bitten by mosquitoes.

A vaccine is now available which is still under trial. Travellers who will be working or travelling for considerable periods in infected areas may be considered for immunization by making enquiries at U.S. Embassies in countries where the disease is endemic.

## TYPHUS FEVER

Epidemic typhus is caused by *Rickettsia prowazekii*, which is transmitted from man to man by the body louse *Pediculus humanis corporis*. Man is the only reservoir of this rickettsia and he becomes infected by rubbing crushed infected lice or their faeces into wounds made by the bites of lice or into other abrasions. Infection may also occur by inhalation of dust contaminated by dried infected louse faeces.

## Vaccine

The vaccine is prepared from formalin-inactivated *R. prowazekii* grown in embryonated eggs and is usually given as two primary subcutaneous injections 7-10 days apart and a reinforcing dose several months later followed by boosters at yearly intervals.

The vaccine is not recommended for travellers staying in urban accommodation in endemic countries. It could be of value to those who expect to be living in close personal contact with the indigenous population of places where the disease occurs, e.g. the mountainous areas of Ethiopia, Rwanda, Burundi, Mexico, Ecuador, Bolivia, Peru and parts of Asia. However, antibiotics are an effective alternative and this vaccine is less frequently used than in the past; it has been withdrawn in the UK but is available elsewhere.

# PLAGUE

Plague is caused by a bacterium *Yersinia pestis* which causes an enzootic infection in wild rodents and other animals in many parts of the world including western USA, South America, south-eastern Russia and parts of Asia and Africa. Direct transmission from rodents or other animals to man may occur in rural areas but the usual method of spread is by fleas, and if the domestic rat population becomes infected epidemics may occur through transmission by fleas of which *Xenopsylla cheopis* is the most important. In the past plague has caused extensive human pandemics with direct person-to-person spread, but at the present time outbreaks in man seem to be limited to Vietnam, Cambodia and Laos, partly as a result of efficient control measures elsewhere but also because of a natural decline of the disease.

## The vaccine

There is a vaccine prepared by inactivating *Y. pestis* with formalin. It is not generally recommended for travellers visiting endemic countries with the exception of Vietnam, Cambodia and Laos, unless their vocation or fieldwork brings them into contact with wild rodents. It is recommended for laboratory personnel working with *Y. pestis* resistant to antimicrobials.

The vaccine should be given intramuscularly in two or three spaced doses with boosters every 6–12 months while the individual remains in the endemic area. While this vaccine can reduce the severity of the disease resulting from contact with infected fleas, the degree of protection against spread by the airborne route is not known.

## MENINGOCOCCAL MENINGITIS

A recent outbreak of meningococcal meningitis among trecker tourists in Nepal with several deaths emphasizes the importance of seeking up-to-date information on prevalent diseases in out of the way places. At the time of writing it is prudent for all travellers to Nepal to be immunized with meningococcal vaccine (see page 131) – but things will change.

# RABIES

Rabies is caused by a rhabdovirus (*rhabdos*, Greek = rod or bullet) and belongs to the *Lyssavirus* genus (*lyssa*, Greek = frenzy). Only one antigenic type of the virus is known. It may be propagated in a wide variety of animals and in tissue cultures. The diagnosis of rabies is based on the finding of cytoplasmic inclusions (Negri bodies) in the brain cells of infected animals or man. (After the bite of an animal (in an endemic country) the animal (usually dog or cat) should be isolated for 10 days and if signs suggestive of rabies develop it should be killed and the brain examined for Negri bodies.)

There are a variety of attenuated virus vaccines for rabies, the concept for which and indeed for all attenuated virus vaccine was initiated by Pasteur 100 years ago with his laboratory-attenuated 'fixed virus' of lower pathogenicity than the natural 'street virus' strains. Immunoprophylaxis is also used.

## The disease

The disease in dogs and cats is similar and is divided into a prodromal, excitative and paralytic phase. In the prodromal stage the animal may show a change in temperament and then during the excitative stage it becomes restless and nervous and wanders about with irritable and vicious tendencies and will bite anything ('furious rabies'): this stage may be very short or absent ('dumb rabies') and is followed by paralysis and death. In cattle, horses etc, the animals become aggressive and 'furious'.

The disease in man is marked by prodromal symptoms of headache, malaise and very often a sensation of tingling, pain or burning around the site of the bite. As the disease progresses excitability and anxiety increase with sensory reactions and hyperaesthesia, and hydrophobia ('fear of water') develops – this being due to the painful spasms of the pharyngeal muscles which arise when attempts are made to swallow fluids. There may be fear of swallowing anything, even the patient's own saliva. Excitation may alternate with periods of relaxation and lucidity and death follows during a period of excitability or following generalized paralysis.

## Epidemiology

Rabies is widely prevalent among various animal species throughout the world. The UK, Ireland, Scandinavia, Spain, Portugal, Cyprus, Australia, New Zealand, Hawaii and other Pacific islands, and parts of the West Indies are free of the disease.

The important animal reservoir in Europe includes foxes, badgers and wolves. In Africa it is the mongoose and jackal; in the Americas the skunk, fox, racoon and fruit-eating bat; in Trinidad and South and Central America it is the vampire bat. (Other animal hosts are stoats, monkeys, deer and cattle which are essentially dead-end hosts.) Rural rabies is a disease of wild biting animals, with sporadic disease among dogs and domestic animals. In urban rabies, dogs are the most important source of infection for man.

Although there were over 55 000 cases of animal rabies reported in Europe between 1979 and 1981, there were only nine human cases. The virus is present in high titre in the saliva, and man usually becomes infected by the bite of an infected animal, but contact by licking may also transmit the disease. The incubation period depends on the site and also on the severity of the bite which determines the dose of virus introduced. The incubation period may be a few weeks after bites of the face and head but up to 6 months after bites of the extremities.

In recent years wildlife rabies has been steadily increasing in the USA. In the UK, apart from two separate importations in monkeys in 1969 and 1970, there has been no animal rabies outside animal quarantine kennels for many years. The few fatal cases in man have all been infected abroad.

## Control

This depends primarily on control of the animal hosts and vaccination of dogs in endemic countries.

## Prevention in man

Travellers in countries where rabies is present should avoid contact with wild animals and with domestic pets. This applies particularly to dogs and cats. Stray animals around camp sites (including puppies and kittens) should be avoided; docile and friendly animals may be suffering from 'dumb' rabies.

If an individual is bitten the wound should be washed with soap and water. If the owner of the suspected animal can be identified, information should be sought on its vaccination status because recently vaccinated animals rarely transmit rabies. In any event, immediate medical advice should be obtained locally because the biting species may be known *not* to be infected, but if so, the local doctor should be able to advise on immunization. If no diploid vaccine is available, the bitten individual should return to the UK or other home base where this vaccine *will* be available.

## Vaccine

Pasteur and rabies vaccine are practically synonymous and up until recently the most widely used modification of the Pasteur vaccine was inactivated rabbit-brain-virus-vaccine developed by Semple. Because of 'neuroparalytic accidents' following administration of this type of vaccine, efforts were made to remove the encephalitogenic allergen by extracting the myelin with arcton. Vaccines were also developed by growing the virus in duck eggs, and duck embryo vaccine (DEV) appeared to produce fewer cases of allergic encephalitis, but it is less antigenic than the Semple vaccine. The factor producing allergic encephalitis appears to be absent from the brains of suckling mice less than 12 days old, and an inactive suckling mouse-brain-virus vaccine (SNBV) has been used extensively in South America and in the USSR.

The vaccine of choice at present is an inactivated vaccine prepared in human diploid cell culture (HDCV). Preliminary studies at the Institut Pasteur of a fetal bovine kidney cell vaccine look promising.

## Pre-exposure vaccination

Vaccination is recommended for those working in quarantine stations, veterinary surgeons, animal handlers, and travellers at high risk of contact with wild animals and bats. (This does not mean that post-exposure immunization can be omitted in the event of a known exposure of such immunized individuals.) The vaccine of choice is HDCV which was originally recommended in a dose of 1.0 ml given intramuscularly on days 0, 7 and 21 or 28. The dosage required is still under review. It appears that a dose of 0.1 ml given intradermally at these intervals, or two doses of 0.1 ml given intradermally at 4-week intervals and a booster at 1 year are acceptable alternatives. Boosters every 2 years should be given to persons at continuing high risk or at shorter intervals to laboratory workers, depending on their levels of rabies antibody.

## Reactions

Redness and slight induration may occasionally occur at the site of the injection and mild fever for a couple of days. Neuroparalytic reactions have not been reported with HDCV and there are no known special contraindications.

## Treatment of wounds

The local treatment recommended by WHO for wounds involving possible exposure is as follows:

(1) *First-aid treatment:* 'Since elimination of rabies virus at the site of infection by chemical or physical means is the most effective mechanism of protection, immediate washing and flushing with soap and water, detergent, or water alone is imperative (recommended procedure in all bite wounds including those unrelated to possible exposure to rabies). Then apply either 40–70% alcohol, tincture or aqueous solutions of iodine, or 0.1% quaternary ammonium compounds.' (Where soap has been used to clean wounds, all trace of it should be removed before the application of quaternary ammonium compounds because soap neutralizes the activity of such compounds.)

(2) *'Treatment by or under direction of a physician*
   (a) Treat as above and then:
   (b) Apply antirabies serum by careful instillation in the depth of the wound and by infiltration around the wound.
   (c) Postpone suturing of wound; if suturing is necessary use antiserum locally as stated above.
   (d) Where indicated, institute antitetanus procedures and administer antibiotics and drugs to control infections other than rabies.'

## Postexposure treatment

Postexposure immunization is practical because of the long incubation period which usually follows infection, for the virus undergoes a period of local multiplication in muscle before spreading to the c.n.s. by way of peripheral nerves.

Postexposure active immunization may be accompanied by passive immunization. The usual antiserum available is equine in origin and the dosage is 40 iu/kg bodyweight. This may give rise to allergic reactions and it is better to use specific rabies human immunoglobulin in a dose of 20 iu/kg which is free from reactions.

## Administration of the vaccine

The postexposure schedule for HDCV recommended by the manufacturer (Merieux) is 1 ml vaccine subcutaneously on day 0, 3, 7, 14 30 and 90. There is increasing evidence that the intradermal (i.d.) route of administration is more efficient and obviously more economical. Multi-site (i.d.) schedules such as 0.1 ml × 8 (day 0), 0.1 ml × 4 (day 7), 0.1 ml (days 28 and 91) or 0.1 ml × 4 (day 1) and 0.1 ml on days 2, 4, 6, 13 and 29 appear to be very effective.

The best specific treatment is combined serum and vaccine therapy and the serum is usually given as a single dose at the same time as the first dose of vaccine but at another site: serum may be given 24 hours before commencing the vaccine course.

Where a reliable history is not available it is justifiable to modify the course and give a single dose of serum and three daily doses of vaccine. Provided the suspected animal stays healthy for 10 days, no further vaccine should be required (see Table 21).

## Evaluation of vaccine

Each year about a million people throughout the world are given courses of rabies vaccines, but controlled studies of its effectiveness have never been made. One study in India using Semple vaccine indicated that 56% of untreated exposed individuals developed rabies compared with 7% who had been vaccinated. Comparable figures are not available for the HDCV but greatly enhanced protection can be anticipated because of the much greater antigenicity of the vaccine as measured by antibody production.

**Table 21** Specific systemic treatment (WHO recommendations)

| Nature of exposure | Status of biting animal | | Recommended treatment |
| --- | --- | --- | --- |
| | At time of exposure | During 10 days* | |
| 1. Contact but no lesions, indirect contact, no contact | Rabid | | None |
| 2. Licks of the skin, scratches or abrasions, minor bites (covered areas of arms, trunk, and legs) | (a) Suspected as rabid† | Healthy | Start vaccine. Stop treatment if animal remains healthy for 5 days*,‡. |
| | | Rabid | Start vaccine, administer serum upon positive diagnosis and complete the course of vaccine |
| | (b) Rabid, wild animal§, or animal unavailable for observation | | Serum + vaccine |
| 3. Licks of mucosa, major bites (multiple or on face, head, finger or neck) | Suspect† or rabid domestic or wild§ animal, or animal unavailable for observation | | Serum + vaccine. Stop treatment if animal remains healthy for 5 days*‡ |

* Observation period in this chart applies only to dogs and cats. Wild life should be killed and examined immediately because the incubation period in many wild animals may be very long
† All unprovoked bites in endemic areas should be considered suspect unless proved negative by laboratory examination
‡ Or if its brain is found negative by fluorescent antibody examination
§ In general, exposure to rodents and rabbits seldom, if ever, requires specific antirabies treatment

# 12
# Immunization in Developing Countries

There is a great deal of literature available on this subject from WHO (The Expanded Programme of Immunisation) and also from a number of non-governmental organizations and this chapter is merely a resumé of what I think are the more important aspects of the problem.

Infectious diseases are priority causes of morbidity and mortality in developing countries. Vaccines are no substitute for general improvements in socioeconomic conditions in their prevention and control. Even with the most advanced medical technology, immunization by itself is unlikely to compensate for adverse effects of environmental and behavioural factors. It will produce poor and disappointing results *unless* it is accompanied by: control of the source of infection; breaking the chain of transmission; increasing the resistance of the host.

## Immunization programmes

Obviously, the first requirement is to know something about the incidence of the various diseases and their age specific attack rates in order to identify the target population to be immunized. In developing countries this information often comes from two sources: (1) what governments consider are their main health problems (which is often based on impressions), (2) the reported causes of death, and (3) hospital and clinic attendances. In some countries this information may not even include the diseases for which some vaccines are available.

Basic epidemiological data are required to define the size of the problem and so that immunization programmes may be planned for the target population. It is not possible to extrapolate from one disease or from one country to another.

It has been estimated that in developing countries of every 1000 children born, 'five will grow up crippled with poliomyelitis, ten die of neonatal tetanus, 20 die of whooping cough (pertussis) and 30 or more die of measles or its complications'. During 1984, measles, pertussis, tetanus, poliomyelitis, diphtheria and tuberculosis were responsible for the death of 4 million children in the world and these diseases caused an additional 4 million children to become physically or mentally handicapped.

## Socioeconomic conditions

While the vaccine preventible diseases are priority causes of morbidity and mortality it must not be forgotten that over the years, long before there were any vaccines available in the UK or in other (now) developed countries, the decline in whooping cough, measles and tuberculosis was dependent on better social conditions, smaller family size and the reduction of overcrowding, better housing, better nutrition and improvements in public health. In developing countries the importance of improved environmental conditions, family planning and health education must not take second place to the introduction of immunization programmes. They must not be introduced in isolation but should be developed as part of a programme of primary health care (PHC) 'within the structure of the development of an appropriate and equitable care infrastructure, involving the community and sectors other than health' which have an impact on the well-being of the people in that community (Alma Ata, WHO, UNICEF, 1978).

## The Expanded Programme of Immunization (EPI)

In May 1974, the 27th WHO World Health Assembly promulgated a resolution committing WHO to the Expanded Programme of Immunization (EPI) which was set up with the objective of reducing morbidity and mortality from diphtheria, pertussis, tetanus, measles, poliomyelitis and tuberculosis by providing immunization against these diseases for all children of the world by 1990. While these diseases have by now been largely eliminated from many parts of the developed world, very many children living in underdeveloped countries are still awaiting immunization against them. Not only are these children susceptible to infection with these diseases but they are liable to a more serious outcome if they become infected – e.g. in measles, malnutrition produces an increased mortality; in poliomyelitis the absence of rehabilitation leads to more crippling of those who survive.

These six diseases are worldwide in distribution and for most of them relatively cheap vaccines are available to prevent them, but there are many problems in making them available to all who require them.

Any immunization programme will in the first place need political support and adequate resources. EPI has been particularly effective in the organizational and administrative side in developing and implementing the technique of 'cluster' sampling of the target population to determine the prevalence of the six diseases, in making vaccines available, in ensuring that the quality is satisfactory, in advising on coverage, in the development of the 'cold chain' so essential for the transport of poliomyelitis and measles vaccines, in training health care workers and in helping to establish personnel with adequate management and organization skills.

In setting up an immunization programme it is essential to involve the local community. Consideration must be given to what the community wants and needs and will actively support. In part this must be based on their beliefs and culture and much effort may be required to establish confidence in the immunization programme and to ensure that its advantages become obvious.

In developing countries the urban immunization programmes will have similar schedules of immunization to those in developed countries, but needs of rural communities cannot be extrapolated from urban data.

In most situations the technology of vaccine dosage and schedules has been transported from the rich to the poor without considering that different dosages and schedules will probably be required and only recently has consideration been given to modifying the schedules to the needs of children in the developing subtropical and tropical world (see Table 23).

In general there are basically three strategies for providing immunization services in developing countries and their relative advantages and disadvantages are outlined in Table 22.

In developed countries, vaccination programmes have been pre-dominantly based on static health facilities. In developing countries, where it is usually much more difficult for people to attend static services (for a variety of physical, infrastructural, cultural and moti-vational reasons), it is likely that improved coverage will depend on making more effort to take the services to the people. Outreach

**Table 22**  Immunization service strategies for developing countries*

| Type of immunization service | | |
|---|---|---|
| Static (e.g. clinic and other health facilities) | Outreach (e.g. satellite services and mobile PHC teams) | Mass campaigns (e.g. single vaccine total coverage (polio); all vaccines offered according to need) |
| *Advantages* Other PHC services and health records are readily available | Takes the services to the people (therefore, relies less on people's motivation) | High coverage possible provided there is good planning and promotion, 'national commitment', intersectoral co-operation and community participation |
| Easier to link immunization and other PHC activities – for staff and community | Some other PHC activities could be provided at the same time | |
| Unnecessary for staff to travel (which decreases costs and inconvenience to staff) | Helps health workers to get to know their communities | High quality vaccination service possible with adequate training |
| Supervision and in-service training are easier | | In some circumstances costs may be cheaper than alternative approaches |
| | | Useful short term measure (whilst the PHC infrastructure is being developed) |
| | | Advantages likely to be greatest in areas of lowest coverage: useful for very dispersed populations |

**Table 22**—*continued*

|  | *Type of immunization service* | |
| --- | --- | --- |
| *Static (e.g. clinic and other health facilities)* | *Outreach (e.g. satellite services and mobile PHC teams)* | *Mass campaigns (e.g. single vaccine total coverage (polio); all vaccines offered according to need)* |
| *Disadvantages* | | |
| Success depends on the community's willingness and ability to use the service (e.g. transport, clinic hours) | Necessitates travel and per diem costs for staff | Discontinuation or disruption of other PHC and health-related activities (during the planning and implementation phases) |
| Attendance likely to be affected both positively and negatively, by the quality of the other services which are provided from these health facilities | Increased inconvenience for staff Supervision more difficult Equipment and records less likely to be available | |
| | | Must be continued every year until the infrastructure can cope with routine immunization on demand |
| Difficult to obtain good coverage until there have been significant infrastructural developments | May be vaccine wastage Small numbers of people are contacted only | It may be difficult to maintain the enthusiasm which is necessary for the success of mass programmes |
| Costs may be high if the population density is low | The cold chain is more difficult to maintain | Requires major inter-sectoral co-operation (e.g. schools, transport, media etc) |

*From Dick, B. (1985). Issues in immunization in developing countries. Evaluation and Planning Centre for Health Care, Publ. 7, London School of Hygiene and Tropical Medicine

programmes are most likely to be able to improve the accessibility of the services whilst at the same time developing immunization services within the overall framework of PHC.

'Although mass campaigns may achieve high coverage rates, they are, of necessity, based on a vertical rather than an integrated approach to health care delivery. Certainly, they can achieve impressive results, although whether these can be maintained remains to be seen. If linked to basic infrastructural health care developments they may be an appropriate short term measure for decreasing mortality and morbidity. However, they would seem to be an inappropriate long-term measure in countries which have adopted PHC policies. There is also very little known about the disruptive effects of such programmes on other health services or about the opportunity costs both financial and otherwise, which may result from the diversion of resources from other routine activities.

'None of the strategies outlined (in Table 22) are as clear cut as they might appear and there are many variations on these basic themes. For example, mass campaigns may include one vaccine or the full range of vaccines, they may provide total coverage for the target group or may merely be directed to susceptible children, and they may be provided in combination with routine services or as "catch-up" or "pulse" programmes. An additional decision which needs to be taken for certain outreach strategies and mass campaigns generally, is whether people should be immunized on a home-to-home basis or whether they should come to a centralized collecting point. This decision will be affected by a number of factors including the cultural characteristics of the communities, population density and cost. For static health facilities, decisions will need to be taken as to whether immunization will be available routinely, on demand, or whether it will only be available on certain days.

'In the same way that decisions about strategies will depend on other policy decisions in the health sector and on a number of epidemiological and economic considerations, choices about who actually administers the vaccines will depend on the choice of strategy. If a mass campaign approach is adopted then it is unrealistic to expect the PHC workers to carry out all the immunizations. If immunization services are provided from static facilities then there would be obvious advantages if the PHC workers were responsible for immunization as well as for the other PHC activities. However, this will depend on their ability to accept additional responsibilities. It will also depend on whether the additional training, supervision and logistic support can be justified by the potential number of people who might be vaccinated' (Bruce Dick, 1985).

Developments along these lines, largely initiated and sponsored by EPI and non-governmental organizations such as Save the Children

Fund, have produced quite remarkable results in working towards the goal of 'Health for all by 2000'.

## Tuberculosis

Although there is a continuing debate on the efficiency of BCG in both developing and developed countries, there seems to be little doubt that potent BCG vaccines are effective in preventing miliary tuberculosis and tuberculosis meningitis in children. The action to be taken in regard to BCG will vary from country to country and will depend on its efficiency and cost-effectiveness. In those countries where tuber-culosis rates are high, where health care facilities are remote and health care personnel limited, if there is an existing BCG programme, it would seem sensible to continue it and to graft other routine immu-nization programmes onto it and expand it throughout the country.

In countries such as Uganda, where a more than 80% protection against both tuberculosis and leprosy was claimed from BCG immu-nization, it was estimated that the cost of treating a tuberculous child in hospital could provide BCG immunization of 7000 individuals.

## Diphtheria (dip/tet/pert and plus typhoid)

Dip/tet/pert/(the triple antigen) is a simple and cheap vaccine to manufacture and administer.

The prevalence of diphtheria as a nasopharyngeal infection seems to be relatively infrequent in tropical countries where diphtheria skin infections are more frequent. These infections are presumably asso-ciated with the production of antitoxin giving protection against the classical type of infection; this may change as a country becomes more developed. The prevalence of pertussis is said to be high in developing countries but, like diphtheria and tetanus, this is not well documented. The tetanus component provides a basic immunity for boosters (see page 166). Tetanus toxoid by itself is of importance in the prevention of neonatal tetanus (see below).

In countries with a high incidence of enteric fever, typhoid vaccines could be combined dip/tet/pert as boosters for older children. (In order to avoid reactions about one third of the recommended dose could be given intradermally (i.d.): it will give the same antibody responses as dip/tet/pertussis and typhoid vaccines given subcutaneously. Not only would this reduce reactions to the typhoid component but also it provides a useful marker for some weeks at the site of inoculation; however, skill is required to ensure that the dose is given i.d.)

The use of typhoid vaccine should not be allowed to vitiate efforts to provide pure water and health education.

## Neonatal tetanus

This condition is caused by the contamination of the umbilical stump with *Cl. tetani* as a result of cutting the cord with unsterilized instruments and/or using dirty cloth or other material contaminated with animal excreta or soil containing tetanus spores as a dressing, or root strings to tie the cord.

Neonatal tetanus is associated with spasm of the muscles and rigidity of the body of the baby. The first sign of infection is usually failure to suck by a baby who has sucked normally for the first few days after birth. It is nearly always fatal in the first week of life but death may not occur until up to the fourth week. In most developing countries the total number of neonatal deaths from all causes varies from about 20 to 30 per 1000 live births, but is very much higher in some places. Of these deaths one quarter to three quarters are due to neonatal tetanus and, excluding China, up to 1 million babies are lost each year due to this condition. In some parts of the world neonatal tetanus is so frequent that it is accepted as a natural hazard of childbirth.

Prevention depends in the first place on the education of mothers and birth attendants in hygienic delivery practices and in providing where possible a sterile cutting instrument and a simple ointment to dress the umbilicus rather than clay, herbs, honey or animal excreta. The second arm of prevention is immunization. If a girl has been immunized with dip/tet/pert vaccine as a baby and given reinforcing doses at suitable intervals, her baby will have maternal antibody and immunity to tetanus to transmit to her baby at birth. Otherwise women who have not been immunized in childhood should be immunized during their first pregnancy with two doses of vaccine and given reinforcing doses (see page 34). The strategy of immunization for mothers will vary from country to country depending on the co-operation of maternal and child welfare clinics and PHC in general in the immunization programmes. It is important that, as part of the immunization programme for neonatal tetanus, data are collected on its incidence and of the efficiency of the immunization programme if for nothing else than to boost health education.

## Poliomyelitis

In the past, many health administrators did not consider that polio-myelitis was a priority disease in tropical countries but the falseness of that impression was shown by the results of 'lameness surveys' introduced in the EPI. From these studies it could be estimated that there were more than a million children in the world crippled by polio-myelitis and several studies have shown that under varying conditions poliovirus vaccine is cost-effective.

The reason for the frequency of poliomyelitis in small children in developing countries is largely the increased opportunities for faecal-oral transmission of the virus, but perhaps also it results from low levels of maternal antibody. Although there are no data to support the suggestion that the lower rates of antibody conversion following immunization with OPV in babies in some tropical countries is because of their poor nutritional state, while the response to some antigens such as yellow fever virus is impaired in malnourished children. Antibody which has developed in girls following infection in childhood may never reach a very high level. When such girls have babies, the maternal antibody which they transmit may be of such low titre that it rapidly falls below an effective protective level. The baby is then susceptible to poliomyelitis in the first few months of life as compared with babies in other parts of the world, who in the more recent pre-immunization days probably had maternal antibody for a considerable time during the first year of life. There is evidence that the pattern of antibody response is much better if a baby is breast fed or fed high protein cow's milk, and poorer with low protein cow's milk or soya bean formula.

Oral poliovirus vaccine (OPV) has been more extensively used than inactivated poliovirus vaccines (IPV) but, with cheaper ways of making potent IPV, with a reduction of the number of doses to two and perhaps even to one and with the proven efficiency of combined quadruple polio/dip/tet/pert vaccine, the attractiveness of IPV is increasing; but furthermore, for as yet unknown reasons, OPV is less effective than IPV in tropical and subtropical countries (as measured by the levels of circulating antibodies). There is no good evidence that interference by other enteroviruses is of special importance in this respect, nor that breast milk influences vaccine 'takes'. (The suggestion that breast feeding should be withheld 6 hours prior to and following a dose of OPV because of the supposed inhibitory effect of milk on the viruses is not supported by laboratory studies.)

OPV and measles vaccines are readily inactivated at temperatures above 4°C. This has meant that these vaccines have had to be kept cold from the time they are manufactured to the time that they are administered. This has been achieved often with great difficulty under field conditions by the 'cold chain' of fridges and cold boxes. Failure of the 'cold chain' has often meant that the vaccine administered has been incapable of stimulating antibody production. Stabilizers have now been added to some vaccines, which has increased their thermostability, and heat sensitive indicators have been produced to provide evidence of the maintenance of low temperatures during transport.

It must be ensured that all vaccines made available for immunization programmes in developing countries comply in all details with the WHO requirements. As with all vaccines there must be continuous surveillance. It would seem more sensible to base studies on the efficacy of poliovirus vaccines on paralytic attack rates than on antibody surveys.

## Measles

In some developing countries measles is the commonest infectious disease in children and its severity is related to their state of nutrition. In developed countries measles has its highest attack rates in 3–5-year-old children but in the underdeveloped world it is in the 1–2-year age group, with the highest mortality in the under-1-year-olds. It is a major (sometimes *the* major) cause of death in children between the ages of 1 and 4 years in the Third World, complicated by diarrhoea, dehydration and bronchopneumonia, and the associated malnutrition with vitamin A deficiency in those who survive often leads to blindness, for the cornea 'melts away'. It is not the virus which makes the mortality in a malnourished child 400 times greater than in a well-nourished one but the diet and the culture of the community. In some places the mortality from measles closely parallels that of kwashiorkor, and measles is probably the commonest precipitating factor of protein malnutrition. Reduction of malnutrition could have a very great effect on measles mortality and reduction of measles would reduce the effects of malnutrition.

More mistakes have been made in measles vaccination programmes than have been seen with any other vaccine; no programme should be started without consideration of the long-range implications of its introduction; and immunization against measles must be integrated, with other immunizations, with health education, maternal and child welfare and family planning programmes. Because of the younger age of infection of measles and of the high birth rate in developing countries, immunization against measles should, as far as possible, be carried out at about 9 months of age.

With the development of stabilizers resulting in less rigid 'cold chain' requirements measles vaccine should become less expensive to store and to deliver. An example of the problem of cost was highlighted in data from an analysis of a measles immunization campaign in the Cameroons some years ago. This showed that 83% of the vaccine which was delivered was wasted, 44% of the children were immune to measles, 1.4% were too young or too old at the time of the campaign, 25% of the vaccine administered was impotent because of loss of titre due to tropical conditions and 12.6% of the vaccine was thrown away. An effective inactivated measles vaccine could be a great advantage and perhaps in the future a polyvalent inactivated virus mixture might, in a single shot, immunize against the majority of common childhood diseases.

## Schedules of immunization

In 1984, 60 million children reached 1 year of age in the developing world; very little work seems to be in progress to establish the optimum schedules and age for their immunization. Those which have often been recommended in recent years have usually followed those which are used in Europe and in North America, with little rationale except that they were effective, and without always appreciating that the epidemiology of diseases varies from country to country. In establishing any schedule it is desirable to immunize the individual just before the age of highest morbidity of the disease. This can be more readily and accurately ascertained by information on age-specific attack rates than by serological tests. In general, since most infectious diseases

**Table 23** Characteristics of vaccines included in the Expanded Programme on Immunization (after EPI, WHO)

| Vaccine | Number of doses | Start of immunization | Intervals between doses | Route of administration | Stability at 37 °C (approx.) |
|---|---|---|---|---|---|
| Measles | 1 | 9 months + (12–15 months) | — | s.c. or i.m.[1] | 7, (30)[2] days |
| BCG | 1 | From birth | — | i.d.[1] | 7 days |
| DPT | 3<br>2[3] | From 6 weeks[4]<br>at 4–6 months[4] | 4 weeks | s.c. or i.m. | 7 days |
| OPV | 3[4] | From 6 weeks<br>at birth[5] | 4 weeks | oral | 1 day |
| IPV[6] | 2 | From 3 months | 4–6 months | s.c. or i.m. | 7 days |
| T | 2<br>1 | Adult primary course<br>Booster | 4 weeks<br>during pregnancy | s.c. or i.m. | 2 months |

[1] s.c. = deep subcutaneous; i.m. = intermuscular; i.d. = intradermal
[2] if modern vaccine adequately stabilized
[3] may suffice if high potency vaccine
[4] an additional dose frequently given during second year of life
[5] needs further evaluation
[6] single dose and earlier starting being evaluated

occur at an earlier age in developing countries than in industrialized ones, the age for commencing immunization in the former should be younger (Table 23).

## Surveillance

Surveillance is all-important and the data collected should not just be filed! They must be used to evaluate the efficiency and the cost-effectiveness of the programme and to modify it or expand it as indicated. If surveillance of a disease is to be successful it must lead to action.

## Addendum

### Immunizations save 800 000 infants' lives in the developing world

An estimated 800 000 infants' lives are saved each year in developing countries by immunizations against 6 childhood diseases – polio-myelitis, diphtheria, pertussis, tetanus, measles and tuberculosis – by 1990 60–70% of all infants in developing countries will receive immunizations. Despite these successes, however, an estimated 265 000 cases of poliomyelitis, 2 million deaths from measles and 600 000 deaths from pertussis still occur each year in the developing world (WHO, 1985).

# 13
# Passive Immunization

It will be recalled that with passive immunization, immunity is achieved by injecting antibodies from another host. The onset of the protection is immediate and its duration depends on the titre of antibodies in the donor serum. Passive immunization may be used therapeutically to provide protection until the host has developed antibodies as a result of immunization or a natural infection, or to prevent an infection for which active immunization is neither indicated nor available.

## Natural passive immunity

In the case of natural passive immunity, IgG is transferred across the placenta from plasma of the mother and the IgG is normally broken down with a half-life of about 3–4 weeks. For all practical purposes the duration of protection is about 6–9 months in normal babies. In premature infants the transferred antibody may be below the level which will protect; it may be augmented artificially by the injection of immunoglobulins. (IgM does not pass the placental barrier and IgA is found essentially on serous surfaces and in colostrum and is protective against invasion of these surfaces.)

## Artificial passive immunity

In artificial passive immunity the injection of immunoglobulins which contain 90% IgG produces immediate protection and there is obviously no lag phase nor any secondary response if further injections of the immunoglobulins are made. In fact, when immunoglobulins from a foreign host are injected they are catabolized like any other protein, or used in reactions with the antigens of the invading organism.

Normally antibodies to foreign immunoglobulins will develop about 10–14 days after injection, but if the host has had previous experience with the foreign immunoglobulin the antibodies to it will develop more quickly and the 'serum' will be rapidly eliminated. This presented a problem when horse antitetanus serum (ATS) was used in the prophylaxis of tetanus, for any repeated injection of horse serum often caused such rapid production of antibody against it that the ATS antitoxin was removed from the circulation and rendered ineffective long before it had had the chance to protect the patient. The combination of horse serum with precipitating antigen in the tissues may lead to serum sickness (hypersensitivity type 3), or to anaphylactic shock (hypersensitivity type 1) and death. These properties of horse and other animal sera led to their virtual abandonment for use in passive immunization and human immunoglobulin has taken their place.

Theoretically, different classes of human immunoglobulins could elicit antigen–antibody reactions, but because they are homologous they do not excite the type of antibody response elicited by foreign animal proteins unless they are inoculated intravenously, when they may produce severe reactions because of aggregations of antibody molecules which react with complement.

Various treatments of immunoglobulin to reduce the amount of aggregated material or limit its biological (phlogistic) activity have been introduced, which does not affect the antigen–combining activity of antibodies, but only their secondary biological functions. These modified immunoglobulins are suitable for intravenous use for conditions such as immunodeficiency. (Recently non-A,non-B hepatitis has been reported in immunodeficient patients given modified intravenous immunoglobulin (IVIG) and this requires investigations.)

## Normal immunoglobulin

The immunoglobulins in common use are prepared from pools of human plasma or placental blood. The immunoglobulin prepared from normal sources was called *gammaglobulin*, but it is now referred to as *human normal immunoglobulin* in Britain and *immune serum globulin (human)* in the USA. In the preparation of human normal immunoglobulin, the plasma from at least 1000 donors is used for each batch; thus all batches will have comparable levels of the antibodies prevalent in the donor community. Protective antibodies to *all* infectious diseases will not be represented in preparations of immuno-globulin, for normal immunoglobulin contains mainly IgG which is not generally effective against *invasive* bacteria. Immunoglobulins are in general of value only in those bacterial diseases which stimulate antitoxins and in virus infections, particularly those which produce a viraemia and to which immunity is largely mediated by circulating antibody.

In the UK normal immunoglobulin is prepared as a 15 g per cent solution in two sizes of vial: 250 mg in 1.7 ml solution, and 750 mg in 5.1 ml solution. Doses are usually prescribed by weight of immuno-globulin. In the USA immune serum globulin contains 165 mg of gammaglobulin per ml, and consists of most of the antibodies in plasma concentrated about 25 times. Doses are given in ml/kg of body weight.

## Specific immunoglobulin

The second type of human immunoglobulin available was in the past referred to as *hyperimmune gammaglobulin* or convalescent gamma-globulin. This contains increased amounts of antibody to specific diseases (e.g. tetanus and hepatitis B virus (HBV)) and is now called *human specific immunoglobulin* in Britain and *special immune serum globulin* in the USA. The specific names of these preparations are, e.g., human antitetanus immunoglobulin in the UK and tetanus immune globulin (human) in the USA. Specific immunoglobulin is prepared by pooling the blood of convalescent patients or by bleeding immunized donors whose antibody has recently been boosted by immunization.

In the UK specific immunoglobulins are prepared as solutions with a protein content of not less than 10 g or more than 15 g per cent. The immunoglobulins are suspended in saline and give a clear yellowish or slightly brown fluid which should be stored at +4 °C. (They may develop a slight turbidity on storage.) They are prepared at the Blood Products Laboratory, Lister Institute of Preventive Medicine (Elstree) and at the Plasma Fraction Centre, Edinburgh. In England and Wales they are available through the Public Health Laboratory Service Laboratories, with the exception of human antitetanus immunoglobulin, which is kept at a number of designated centres and is also obtainable commercially (Imutet BW). In Scotland normal and specific immunoglobulins are available at regional transfusion centres. Two vial sizes are available: 250 mg and 500 mg.

In the USA information on supply may be obtained from CDC, Atlanta, Georgia.

In Britain the supply of specific immunoglobulin depends on the co-operation of general practitioners, and there is need for antivaricella/zoster, antitetanus and to a lesser extent antimumps, antiherpes simplex and antirubella specific immunoglobulins. Patients who have suffered an attack of one of these diseases (except tetanus) in the previous 3 months should be asked to donate some blood, as should any adult who has recently been reimmunized against tetanus. The names and addresses of anyone volunteering to do so should be sent to the director of the local blood transfusion centre. Supplies of these specific immunoglobulins can only be prepared if such donations of blood are forthcoming.

In the USA the specific immunoglobulins contain about 10 to 20 times the levels of antibody in pools of 'normal' donor sera. As with immune serum globulin, doses in the USA are given in ml/kg body weight.

Immunoglobulins which have been treated so as to be suitable for intravenous administration are available commercially.

## Dosage and reactions

When immunoglobulins are injected, the initial concentration of antibody in the preparation becomes diluted by the body fluids of the recipients to a dilution of plasma equal to about 8% of their body weight. Antibodies which are present in the immunoglobulins in low titre could thus be diluted below a level which on theoretical grounds would be expected to be effective. Because of this dilution factor it is obvious that the weight : dose ratio in the use of immunoglobulins is important. Unless specially treated immunoglobulins should always be injected intramuscularly. Reactions are rare although sometimes there is slight pain at the site of injection. Untreated immunoglobulins must *never* be injected intravenously, because this may produce serious reactions such as tachycardia, pallor, a sense of pressure in the chest, pain in the flank and shock.

## Bacterial infections

## Diphtheria

Diphtheria is one of the very few diseases for which antitoxin prepared in animals is still used. The efficacy of this antitoxin and the disappearance of the disease following immunization with toxoid make the study of human antidiphtheria immunoglobulin virtually irrelevant.

Antitoxin prepared in horses (which, early on, became the animals of choice) was introduced by Roux at the Pasteur Institute at the end of the last century after the discovery of passive immunity by Behring and his colleagues in Berlin. Its use probably reduced the case fatality rate of diphtheria from about 40% to less than 10%. It soon became obvious that some measurement of the amount of antibody in the immunoglobulin was required. This led to the whole concept of standardization not only of sera but of other biological fluids and to the subsequent establishment of many international standards.

For therapy, antidiphtheria serum (ADS) has to be given immediately the clinical diagnosis is made and is said to be 100% effective if given within 24 hours of the onset.

As a prophylactic in the control of outbreaks in the UK, ADS has in recent years been confined to its use in closed institutions such as homes for the mentally subnormal where outbreaks should normally be prevented by active immunization and boosting. After a case has been diagnosed in such a home all contacts and any home contacts should be swabbed (nose and throat) and their immunization status investigated by the Schick test. The amount of toxin in the test dose is adequate to boost the immunity of Schick negative individuals. All Schick positive individuals should be given an injection of toxoid in a form such as PTAP (purified toxin adsorbed on aluminium phosphate) and at the same time 500 units of antitoxin. This antitoxin may give rise to general reactions in about 5-8% of individuals. However, when diphtheria was prevalent it was believed that the risk of diphtheria in the non-immunized was greater than the risk of sensitization to horse serum. All contacts should be kept under close surveillance for 3-4 days until the laboratory results on isolations become available. All individuals who are non-immune should be given a second dose of PTAP 4-6 weeks later. There is no experience of how the availability of penicillin and erythromycin might today modify this regimen.

## Reactions

If horse serum or other animal sera are injected, it must be understood that there are no entirely satisfactory tests for hypersensitivity to animal sera. The greatest reliance on the likelihood of a hypersensitivity reaction should be placed on whether or not the individual has previously been given an injection of animal serum, and whether or not there is any personal or family history of allergic conditions. If there is no experience or history of hypersensitivity, an intramuscular injection of the serum may be given and the patient kept under observation for at least 30 minutes (although serum sickness may develop 7–10 days later). If the patient has previously been given animal serum, he should be given a trial dose of 0.2 ml of serum and observed for 30 minutes. If there is no reaction the rest of the dose of serum may be given intramuscularly. If there is a reaction the serum should be given in 0.2 ml volumes by the subcutaneous route at intervals of 30 minutes until the total dose has been injected.

As patients with an allergic history appear to be at greatest risk of developing severe reactions to foreign sera, they should be given 0.2 ml of the serum diluted 1:10 in distilled water subcutaneously and should be kept under observation for 30 minutes. If there is no reaction, 0.2 ml of the undiluted serum may be given subcutaneously, and if there is no subsequent reaction the remainder of the total dose may be given by the intramuscular route. If there is a reaction the remainder of the serum should be given in 0.2 ml volumes half-hourly, preceded by a dose of a quick-acting antihistamine before the injections are started.

At all times adrenaline (1:1000) and hydrocortisone hemisuccinate should be available for immediate use in case a reaction occurs.

The intravenous injection of serum should be limited to hospital practice.

## Tetanus

As already mentioned (Chapter 4) the prevention of tetanus depends on active immunization of all children with tetanus toxoid, with boosters at school entry and at school leaving and further boosters to adults at high risk. The prophylaxis of tetanus in immunized individuals who suffer wounds or burns has also been discussed and, briefly, their basic immunity may be boosted with tetanus toxoid.

Since reactions occur after the use of animal sera, the use of horse serum for the prophylaxis of tetanus was abandoned by many practitioners before human tetanus immunoglobulin (HTIg) became available, and the use of ATS is now essentially of historical interest in developed countries, and it has been replaced by HTIg which is prepared from the plasma of selected donors whose plasma level of tetanus antitoxin has been boosted by a recent dose of toxoid. HTIg may be in relatively short supply in the UK from DHSS sources, but it is also available commercially. In the treatment of clean wounds (with minimal tissue damage sustained in circumstances unlikely to involve contamination with tetanus spores, such as a cut with a razor or by glass), provided that the patient receives medical attention within 6 hours of the trauma, cleansing and suture and an injection of 0.5 ml adsorbed tetanus toxoid should be recommended, with completion of the course of toxoid as required. With other wounds or burns (with the exception of those listed below) it is usually recommended that in addition to tetanus toxoid and adequate cleansing of the wound, penicillin by injection, preferably as a mixture of benzathine, procaine and benzylpenicillin in the proportions of 2:1:1, to cover for at least 4 days should be given and 0.5 ml adsorbed toxoid. *Subsequently, the course of tetanus toxoid should be completed.* For patients sensitive to penicillin, tetracycline in doses of 250 mg 6-hourly for 4 days may be used.

The experts recommend that HTIg should be used selectively in addition to wound toilet, penicillin, etc, and toxoid, for non-immunized persons who have:

(1) sustained a wound or burn more than 6 hours before attending for treatment,

(2) wounds which are likely to be infected with tetanus organisms because of contamination with soil, manure, etc,

(3) wounds which are septic or contain devitalized tissues,

(4) puncture wounds.

The dose is 250 i.u. given intramuscularly and the preparations usually available contain not less than 50 i.u./ml.

## Other sera

Although potent antisera can be prepared in horses against the organisms of gas gangrene (*Clostridium welchii (Cl. perfringens)*,

*Cl. oedematiens* and *Cl. septicum*), they are rarely used in prophylaxis. Similarly, passive immunization with immunoglobulins against the toxins of *Cl. botulinum* seems to have limited value.

## Virus diseases

## Human normal immunoglobulin (IgG)

In addition to containing antibodies to those 'wild' viruses which are circulating in the community, IgG will presumably also contain antibodies to viral antigens contained in commonly used vaccines (assuming that the viral antigens stimulate reasonable levels of durable circulating antibody).

IgG has been shown to be effective for the prevention of measles, hepatitis A and in certain cases of chickenpox. It is of less use in rubella and poliomyelitis.

### *Measles*

IgG should contain not less than 50 i.u. measles antibody per ml. It has been known to modify or prevent measles since the 1940s and was used widely for this purpose before the introduction of measles vaccine.

The problem of *modifying* a natural infection of measles in infants under 6 months of age should not arise unless they are premature since, at present, nearly all normal babies have maternally transmitted measles antibodies which are usually effective for at least the first 6 months of life. The dosage recommended when given not more than 1 week after exposure is 250 mg (0.05 ml/kg body weight in the USA).

For *prevention* of measles the use of immunoglobulin is essentially limited to the few babies in whom an attack of measles must be avoided, e.g. the small chronically ill baby with respiratory or cardiac disease who, if exposed to measles infection, could be tided over the infection and actively immunized at a convenient time. Passive immunization should be attempted as soon as possible after exposure. The recommended dose is 250 mg and for children 1-2 years and 3 years and over, 500 and 750 mg respectively. (The dose in the USA is 0.25 ml/kg of body weight.) This method of prevention decreases in effectiveness the longer the delay after exposure, and after 4 days it is likely that only attenuation of the infection will be achieved.

IgG has also been used to modify the reactions of measles vaccine in children where there are special considerations to avoid reactions such as (1) children whose parents or siblings have a history of idiopathic epilepsy, (2) children with developmental delay due to a neurological disease and (3) children suffering from chronic diseases of the heart or lungs. In the UK supplies for this purpose are held by local authorities. The optimum dose for modification of reactions is about 0.6 mg/lb body weight. Each vial contains 4-8 i.u. measles antibody in 15 mg immunoglobulin (in the form of 0.5 ml of 3 g per cent solution), sufficient for a child in the second year of life. It is important not to exceed this dose because excess immunoglobulin may inhibit the multiplication of measles vaccine virus. The dose of immunoglobulin is given at the same time as the measles vaccine in the opposite limb.

## Hepatitis A virus (HAV)

Many studies have shown the value of normal immunoglobulin in the prevention and control of clinical manifestations of infective hepatitis. It is of particular value in controlling infection in contacts in mental and other closed institutions, such as children's homes, where the risk of spread of the disease is great. It has also been recommended under certain conditions in ordinary schools and in the protection of home contacts, particularly pregnant women.

It should be given as early as possible after exposure but it still appears to prevent the clinical illness if given as late as 14 days after exposure. Individuals who have been passively immunized may develop jaundice within the first 2 weeks after injection of immunoglobulin, presumably because it has been given too late in the incubation period of the infection. It is effective in preventing clinical disease in about 85% of contacts. In the UK the recommended dose is 250 mg for children under 10 years of age and 500 mg for those of 10 years or more. In the USA 0.02 ml/kg body weight is recommended. It is obvious that the use of gammaglobulin in the control of infection among contacts varies greatly from one situation to another and depends on the degree and nature of the contact.

IgG is also recommended for travellers visiting countries where the risk of infection is great, i.e. where hygiene is poor and where there are considerable opportunities for faecal–oral contamination. Such countries are obviously included in the continents of Africa, Asia and South America. Since about 30–50% of adults in the UK will probably have antibody to HAV (see page 119), it is best to have their sera tested before deciding to give them IgG. The recommended dose is 750 mg which usually confers protection for at least 6 months and many individuals may get a subclinical infection under cover of the immunoglobulin which should provide a durable immunity. A susceptible traveller who has no antibody and has never had infective hepatitis should be given a second injection of immunoglobulin after 6 months if he remains in the country where the chance of infection is great.

In the USA, immunoglobulin is not recommended for travellers on ordinary tourist routes for less than 3 months; for longer journeys 0.02 ml/kg body weight is recommended and 0.05 ml/body weight for travellers planning to stay 3 months or more in tropical areas or in developing countries where hepatitis A is common and hygiene poor.

IgG should not be given for at least 2 weeks after immunization with any live virus vaccines and as near as possible to the date of departure.

With greater demands for IgG it would seem sensible to request for screening for all those who may request it.

## Varicella (chickenpox)

Chickenpox can be a severe disease with a 20% mortality in the neonatal period in infants with no maternal antibody. IgG may be of some value in modifying such infections in newborn babies known not to have maternal antibody, and in premature and other abnormal babies under 6 months of age if it is given within 3 days of exposure. It would also seem reasonable to give immunoglobulin to a neonate whose mother had developed chickenpox in the last 2 weeks of pregnancy.

Normal immunoglobulin may also be given for the *attenuation* of chickenpox in eczematous and other ill children, in pregnant women and in patients on steroids or immunosuppressive drugs. It will not *prevent* chickenpox (see below, Specific Antivaricella Immunoglobulin).

## Poliomyelitis

Although human normal immunoglobulin contains antibodies in adequate titre to prevent poliomyelitis, its use is rarely indicated in the control of poliomyelitis in view of the effectiveness of vaccination. In any event, the uncertainty of the time of exposure to infection presents a practical difficulty in its effective use.

## Rubella

Normal immunoglobulin should confer protection against rubella if given before exposure. However, in practice normal immunoglobulin cannot regularly be considered to be of practical value in the prevention of congenital defects in women who have been exposed to rubella during pregnancy. There are two reasons for this. Firstly, patients with rubella may be infectious for about a week before the rash appears, and thus susceptible contacts may be infected and already have a viraemia before it is appreciated that infection has occurred. It is then too late to expect normal immunoglobulin to have any effect. Secondly, it seems that the quantity of antibody to rubella even in a large dose of IgG is insufficient to consistently neutralize the virus. (See below, Specific Rubella Immunoglobulin.)

## ECHO 11

There is good evidence that normal immunoglobulin (in a dose of 250 mg intramuscularly) may be effective in the control of outbreaks of ECHO 11 virus among neonates.

## Human specific viral immunoglobulins
### Rubella

The efficacy of immunoglobulin in rubella depends on the dose and titre of the IgG, the time of administration in relation to the time of exposure and the immune status of the woman. High-titre human rubella immune globulin (HRI) given in high doses within 24 hours of viral exposure has been shown to be effective in preventing viraemia in rubella infections.

The logistical problems of administering (HRI) are considerable; there are also difficulties of preparing it. Further studies are clearly indicated in its use for the prevention of rubella in selected susceptible pregnant women where termination of pregnancy cannot be carried out if infection occurs.

## Hepatitis B virus (HBV)

Specific HBV immunoglobulin is prepared from donors with a high titre of anti-HBVs. The supply is limited in the UK because of the small number of suitable donors. As with HAV, it seems that effective passively administered antibody does not prevent infection but makes it milder (passive–active immunity).

*Indications for use* are as follows.

(1) Adults: *inoculation accidents.* This immunoglobulin should be given intramuscularly in a dose of 0.05–0.07 ml/kg body weight following an accidental inoculation of infected blood or other fluids contaminated with HBV. Danger of infection exists from inoculation by a needle-stick accident, the introduction of the virus into the eye or mouth, the contamination of an abrasion or heavy contamination of intact skin or sexual contact. The average adult dose is 5.0 ml which should be given as soon as possible and preferably with 48 hours of the accident. A specimen of blood should be taken for serology before the immunoglobulin is injected and again subsequently. If the pre-immunization sample is found to be negative for $HB_sAg$ and anti-$HB_s$, then a second dose of immunoglobulin should be given a month later.

(2) *Staff and patients.* Under certain circumstances HBV immunoglobulin should be made available for dialysis staff and patients if HBV appears in a dialysis unit, for the control of an outbreak in a hospital unit and if required it should be available for home dialysis helpers.

(3) *Family contacts.* HBV immunoglobulin should be available to spouses of patients with acute hepatitis B following the regimen outlined under (1) – inoculation accidents.

(4) *Infants.* Babies born to mothers with an acute HBV infection in the last trimester of pregnancy or in the first 3 months of the puerperium are at high risk of infection. The risk of infection of babies who are born to white mothers (who have a carrier rate of 0.1–0.5%) is very low; it is much higher in babies of Asiatics, especially Japanese and Chinese infants, where the parents may have a carrier rate of 10–20%. Babies born to mothers who are carriers of HBV require not only specific HBV immunoglobulin but also a course of vaccines (see page 126).

## Vaccinia

Human antivaccinia immunoglobulin prepared from blood collected 3–4 weeks after revaccination is now only of historical interest. It was used for the prevention and treatment of the complications of smallpox vaccination and for the prevention of smallpox in contacts.

## Varicella and zoster (VZ)

Antivaricella/zoster immunoglobulin (VZIG) prepared from individuals convalescent from chickenpox or herpes zoster might be expected to confer passive immunity more effectively than normal immunoglobulin. In appropriate doses it will usually prevent varicella in a contact if given within 96 hours after intimate exposure to a patient with chickenpox in an infectious state (i.e. from 5 days before the eruption to not more than 6 days after the eruption of the first crop of vesicles). VZIG will have no effect if the symptoms of varicella have become evident. Patients who have a previous history of chickenpox or herpes zoster infection should be immune and do not require VZIG.

The main value of specific VZ immunoglobulin is in individuals with immunological abnormalities, e.g. those being treated with steroids or immunosuppressive drugs and those who have leukaemia or other neoplastic diseases in whom an infection with VZ virus might otherwise be a progressive and fatal disease.

Specific VZ immunoglobulin could also be of value to prevent cross-infection with chickenpox in children's wards and to control and prevent death from neonatal infections with varicella in babies with blood dyscrasias and chronic illnesses. The recommended doses of VZ immunoglobulin are given in Table 24.

**Table 24** Recommended doses of VZIG for chickenpox and herpes zoster

| Age (y) | Dose (mg) |
| --- | --- |
| Under 1 | 500 |
| 1–6 | 1000 |
| 7–14 | 1500 |
| 15 and over | 2000 |

It will always be relatively scarce because it can be prepared only from the plasma of adults convalescent from chickenpox or herpes zoster. Such people are urgently required as donors. So far supplies have been insufficient to assess its value.

## Herpes simplex

The value of specific antiherpes simplex immunoglobulin has not yet been adequately studied because of the shortage of supply. It might be of value for treating some cases of disseminated herpes simplex infections.

## Rabies

Human antirabies immunoglobulin can be prepared only from the blood of those who have been actively immunized against rabies, otherwise animal immune sera are used (see page 157).

## Other conditions

In addition to the possible use of immunoglobulin for premature babies and in antibody deficient syndromes, its use can always be considered for any conditions where antibody production is suppressed or reduced.

## Adverse reactions

Reactions to specified immunoglobulins are rare. Redness and swelling at the injection site may occur in 1% of patients and general malaise in about 1%. Severe reactions such as angioneurotic oedema and anaphylactic shock have been reported in less than 1 in 1000,

## Conclusion

Before passive immunization can be fully exploited those preparing the human immunoglobulins must have the fullest co-operation of physicians to encourage those who have recovered from certain virus diseases or have been recently immunized to donate blood.

# 14
# Smallpox (Variola)

Since the last edition of this book was published, smallpox has been eradicated from the world and the only *variola* virus left lies entombed in the deep freezes of laboratories in Porton (UK), Atlanta (USA), Moscow and Tokyo, and possibly in a cadaver buried somewhere in the permafrost. Vaccination against smallpox is no longer routinely recommended anywhere. A brief summary of the background of the epidemiology of smallpox and of its eradication may shed some light on the possibility of global eradication of other diseases.

## The virus and the disease

Smallpox virus is a large DNA virus of the orthopoxvirus genus: the other members of this genus are *vaccinia*, cowpox, monkeypox, rabbit pox and *ectromelia* (mousepox). *Variola* infects only humans and monkeys; cowpox and monkeypox may rarely infect man, mousepox and rabbit pox never. No reservoir of smallpox other than man has been discovered. All these orthopoxviruses are very resistant and withstand drying for long periods of time.

The incubation period of smallpox is about 12 days (14 days from rash to rash). The onset of the illness was sudden with fever which persisted for 4–6 days but usually abated on the third day when the outcrop (or rash) appeared on the face or upper part of the body. The outcrop developed centrifugally but was regionally homogeneous over the body, going through a macular, papular and vesicular stage and proceeding to crusting at about the ninth day of the illness. There were several varieties of this picture, from haemorrhagic smallpox to mild infections due to *variola minor*, or *variola sine eruptione* and modified smallpox in immunized persons.

Smallpox was usually transmitted by direct face-to-face contact but could also occur by contact with infected clothing, bedding or other materials. The disease was not infectious during the incubation period but with the onset of fever and the replication of virus in the nasopharyngeal mucosa and before the onset of the rash, patients were highly infectious. In a classical infection the patient was confined to bed in the first few days of the illness during the time of high infectivity, so that he was not a danger to the community but only to household and hospital contacts.

There were two types of virus – *variola major* which caused a case fatality rate of 30–50% and *variola minor* causing 'alastrim' which had a less than 1.0% case fatality.

## Epidemiology

Smallpox was endemic throughout the world till October 1977 when the last naturally acquired case occurred (although subsequently there was a laboratory-associated outbreak in Birmingham (England) in 1978). Smallpox had been present in the world since antiquity but it did not seem to have become the dreaded disease in Europe till the 16th century. This could have been due to the introduction of *variola major*. It seems that the transmission of smallpox among the Aztecs, who were wholly susceptible, may have induced a change in the virulence of the virus which not only decimated that nation but provided a virulent virus for export to Europe, where *variola major* was rife towards the end of the 17th century, causing serious outbreaks. Smallpox achieved its maximum mortality in England and Wales towards the end of the 18th century when about 20% of all recorded deaths were stated to be due to the disease. So dread was smallpox, because of the resultant disfigurement and high death rate, that mothers would expose their babies to infection in the hope that if they acquired smallpox when they were young it would be mild. This 'old wives' tale' could be explained by the infection being modified by the protective effect of maternally transmitted specific immunoglobulin. During the 19th century there were numerous outbreaks, but in many of them there was a considerably reduced mortality and towards the end of that century it appeared that *variola minor* was again taking over as the endemic virus. This became very obvious between World Wars I and II. In 1935 smallpox ceased to be an endemic disease in the UK. Although the disease ceased to be endemic, there were about 20 importations of *variola major* between 1935 and 1970 – when the last case of smallpox occurred in the UK, apart from two limited laboratory-associated outbreaks in 1973 and 1978.

## Immunization

Immunization against smallpox had been practised for centuries, e.g. as in China from earliest times, by blowing dried crusts from the skin of a patient into the nose of vaccinees, or – as in many places in the Middle Ages – by taking fluid from a vesicle of a mild case and scratching it through the skin. This method called *'variolation'* was used in Britain in the 1700s and was popularized by Lady Mary Wortley Montagu who had seen it performed in Turkey. The method had a mixed reception in England; it did not appear to control smallpox adequately and it caused some mortality in those who were variolated and could spread person-to-person.

In 1796, Jenner performed his first human-to-human 'experiment' by vaccinating a boy with material from a cowpox lesion on the hand of a milkmaid and subsequently challenging him with virulent smallpox material; the boy's survival led to further 'experiments' using virus passed from arm to arm and the introduction of 'vaccination' with 'humanized' lymph. Was the belief of the apocryphal milkmaid true, when she said 'I cannot take smallpox for I have had cowpox'? Some doubt exists as to the true nature of the virus which Jenner used. Was it really cowpox virus? Was it smallpox virus modified by arm-to-arm passage and much less virulent than the single passage virus used for variolation? Was it *variola* modified by transmission through a cow? Was it a mutant of smallpox or cowpox? or was it a recombinant cowpox–smallpox virus? In any event, variolation was made illegal in England in 1840 and although the introduction of 'vaccination' with 'humanized lymph' had considerable opposition, the vaccination of infants was made compulsory in the UK in 1853 and enforced there in 1871 and in the USA in the following year. Following the introduction of universal vaccination in England there was no dramatic decline in the incidence of smallpox. Better social conditions, the control of vagrants, the establishment of workhouses, the setting up of smallpox hospitals and the surveillance and recording of disease were all playing a highly important part in its control, as did the cessation of variolation, which eliminated one source of smallpox virus.

## The vaccine

At the beginning of this century, the preparation of lymph in the skin of calves became approved. This led to the use of standardization lymph to which glycerine was added in order to reduce bacterial contamination, and 'humanized lymph', with its attendant dangers of contamination and the accidental transfer of smallpox, was soon given up.

The origins of the various strains of calf lymph *vaccinia* virus are uncertain and one of the strains commonly used for the commercial production of vaccine is said to have been derived from a mild case of smallpox in the Franco–Prussian War of 1870-1.

In recent times sheep were used instead of calves as vaccinifers in many laboratories, with an occasional passage of stock virus in rabbit or man in order to maintain its antigenicity and produce high titre vaccines. In the preparation of vaccine lymph, the animal's belly and thorax were washed and shaved and virus applied with a scalpel in a series of parallel superficial incisions. After about 4 days the vesicles which had developed were scraped off and the resulting pulp ground up with glycerol and stored at $-10\,^{\circ}\text{C}$ to reduce the bacterial content. Other methods were subsequently introduced in order to produce bacteriologically sterile standard preparations of lymph including growth of the virus in chick embryos or tissue cultures.

## Contraindications

The contraindications to vaccination (except in outbreak control where there were no absolute contraindications) were similar to those for other live virus vaccines with the addition of septic skin conditions.

## Complications of vaccination

The number and types of complications which occurred in the UK between 1951 and 1970 following smallpox vaccination are shown in Table 25.

All of these, except postvaccinial encephalitis, could probably have been greatly reduced by paying attention to the contraindications to vaccination and not vaccinating babies in the first year of life where complication rates were highest.

**Table 25** The number and types of complications which occurred following smallpox vaccination in the UK between 1951 and 1970

| Complications | No. |
| --- | --- |
| Postvaccinial encephalitis | 40 |
| Contact eczema vaccinatum | 16 |
| Vaccinia gangrenosa | 13 |
| Eczema vaccinatum | 11 |
| Benign generalized vaccinia | 2 |
| Others | 19 |

## Vaccination policies

At the beginning of this century vaccination was compulsory, but the 1905 Vaccination Act made conscientious objections to vaccination much easier. By 1914, partly as a result of that Act, but also because of general lack of enforcement, the number of children vaccinated was below 50% and the decline continued over the years. Compulsory vaccination of infants ended in the UK with the introduction of the National Health Service in 1946. Nevertheless, the majority of physicians and the DHSS recommended that infant vaccination should be assiduously pursued, although between 1951 and 1970 there had been at least 101 deaths from vaccination and only 37 deaths from smallpox. In 1972 there was a sudden change in policy and routine, infant vaccination was no longer recommended in the UK and a similar policy change by the United States Public Health Services occurred in 1971! What had led to these sharp about-turns in national policies?

The debate about abandoning infant vaccination centred around the frequency of complications and death in infants following vaccination and on the decreased risk of importation of smallpox which followed the earlier continuing success of the WHO global control programme.

The opposition of the 'establishment' to stopping infant vaccination was powerful and political. Some argued that if infant vaccination was stopped in Britain we would be 'wide open' to devastating epidemics following an importation. They forgot that with an infant vaccination acceptance rate of 30–40% in the previous decade and a herd immunity of about 5-10%, the UK had been susceptible to epidemic spread from importation for many years (and nothing serious had been done to remedy this!). In any event, contrary to the opinion of Jenner smallpox does not spread rapidly and vaccination does not give lifelong protection, but furthermore, small children were not at high risk of infection following importation, for experience in the UK and in Europe during the previous decade had incriminated the hospital as the setting for most outbreaks. A final objection to the abandonment of infant vaccination came from those who (contrary to the available evidence) maintained that complications of vaccination were commoner in adults than in children.

## Control of outbreaks

Up till the early 1940s an importation of smallpox was a signal for mass vaccination which diverted the activities of the health workers who were trying to control the epidemic and killed people from complications who never need have been vaccinated.

In 1944 it was reported by Bradley and colleagues that, in the absence of mass vaccination, an outbreak (caused by a virulent strain of the virus) could be controlled by selective epidemiological control methods.

This involved quarantining of patients and prompt tracing and selective vaccination and surveillance of known or probable contacts. Vaccination on the first day or so after contact prevented infection, and if it were done within the first few days after contact, the disease was often modified. The reason for this protective effect of vaccination is that immunity to *vaccinia* virus develops more rapidly than to *variola major* virus.

Since contacts are not infectious during the incubation period (Figure 20) they could be kept under surveillance after vaccination.

Some argued that outbreak control could hardly prove to be as effective in an unvaccinated community as in a partially vaccinated one. They forgot that the outbreaks which had occurred in the UK since 1900 had never been related to the proportion of vaccinated persons in the communities concerned and that this had varied from 2% to 75%.

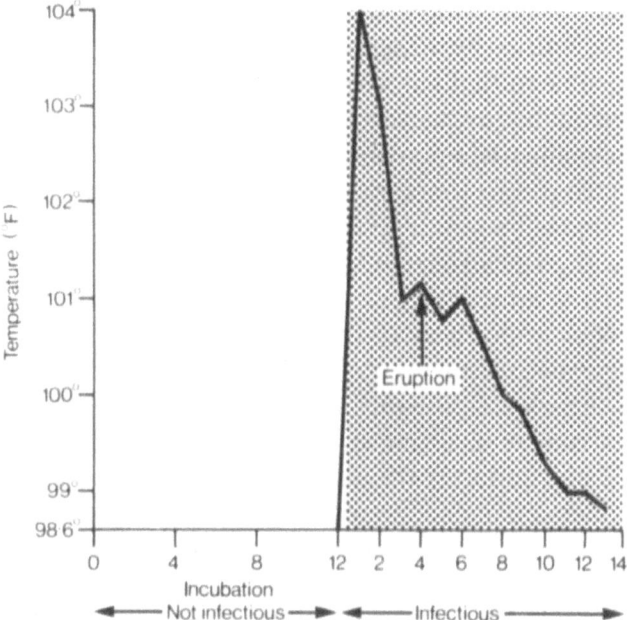

**Figure 20**  Smallpox. Infectious and non-infectious periods

Between 1951 and 1970 there were 13 importations of smallpox into Britain all of which were successfully limited by epidemiological control methods.

If ever there is an escape of smallpox virus from its tombs we know how to control its spread and WHO has arranged that sufficient freeze-dried vaccine to vaccinate 200 million people will be maintained in refrigerated depots in two countries (Switzerland and India) with stocks of bifurcated needles. In addition, 30 countries are individually keeping a total of over 100 million doses of *vaccinia* for their own reserves.

## Global eradication

Early attempts of WHO to control smallpox throughout the world did not succeed for various reasons and it was not till the great powers realized that it was also to *their* advantage to eradicate smallpox that a successful outcome could hopefully be achieved.

The eventual success of the global eradication programme was because (1) it was based on the epidemiological control method described above and not as originally on mass vaccination, (2) patients are readily identified by the outcrop and the scarred faces of survivors made it possible to find out where the cases were (quite a formidable task carried out by roving teams of field workers) and (3) it depended on the development of a preparation of stable freeze-dried vaccine and the bifurcated needle for scarification. An example of the success of this method may be seen, e.g. from experience in West Africa where smallpox was eradicated from Mali and from Sierra Leone which had had the highest attack rates of any country in the world, when only 51% and 66% respectively of the population had been vaccinated – not by mass vaccination.

In 1967 there were probably about 2 500 000 cases of smallpox in the world arising in 42 countries. Thirty of these had endemic small-pox and 12 had imported the disease. By 1973 only four countries – Ethiopia, India, Bangladesh and Pakistan – were considered to be endemic areas and smallpox had been eradicated from South America as indicated by the absence of any cases following 2 years of active surveillance after the discovery of the last known case. In 1974 eradication had been certified in Indonesia, Afghanistan and Pakistan and in Western Africa. At that time Ethiopia remained the only endemic country in the world. By early 1978 smallpox had become limited to a few cases of *variola minor* among nomads along the Ethiopia/Somalia/Kenya borders and in December 1979 the Global Commission of WHO for the Certification of Smallpox Eradication declared the world free of smallpox and recommended that vaccina-tion was no longer required for international travellers, which was soon accepted.

By 1980 the transmission of an infectious disease was interrupted everywhere in the world and the first infectious disease controlled by immunization was eradicated. What about others?

# 15
# New Vaccines

There are a number of new vaccines which have had limited trials and should soon be available for more extensive study.

## Bacterial vaccines

### Burns and wounds

*Pseudomonas aeruginosa* is a Gram-negative non-sporulating bacillus which is a normal commensal in the intestine and skin. It can cause serious infections when it gains entry into tissues devoid of natural defences, e.g. in patients with wounds and burns or with infections of the urinary tract and indeed with many other conditions. It may lead to hospital epidemics among compromised patients. Trials with an inactivated pseudomonas vaccine have been made with some success, sometimes combined with immunotherapy.

### Necrotizing enteritis

A toxoid vaccine from *Clostridium perfringens* type C (*Clostridium welchii*) has considerably reduced death from necrotizing enteritis due to *Cl. perfringens* which is prevalent in children in the highlands of Papua New Guinea.

### Dental caries

A vaccine using a protein from *Streptococcus mutans* has been effective in producing a 70% reduction in dental caries in monkeys.

### Other bacterial diseases

Many other diseases are under study for vaccine development including dysentery, meningitis caused by *Haemophilus influenzae* (type b), leprosy and gonorrhoea (see page 3).

## Virus vaccines

### Chickenpox and shingles

An attenuated varicella virus (OKA) grown in human diploid cells has been tested in normal and in immunosuppressed children and in nurses. It might be used selectively in the latter but further studies are required on its transmissability and stability.

### Japanese B encephalitis virus

A vaccine is now available for selective use (see pages 150–1).

## The future

Many other experimental virus vaccines have provided evidence of their protective efficacy in the laboratory, e.g. Ebola virus (for haemorrhagic fever). Modern technology such as recombinant DNA genetics, the employment of monoclonal antibodies, molecular immunology and immunochemistry will greatly facilitate the production of many new ones. These developments have laid the foundation for a new breed of vaccines, not only for microbial infections but also for vaccines against parasitic infections such as those caused by malaria and schistosoma.

For the future it seems reasonable to assume that the peptides responsible for the development of protective antibodies will be identified and synthesized and used in polyvalent synthetic vaccines or alternatively by incorporating the gene necessary for their production into non-pathogenic viruses or bacteria (by recombinant DNA techniques) it should be to provide replicating non-virulent agents capable of inducing immunity against serious illnesses.

# Index